Advances in
Stroke

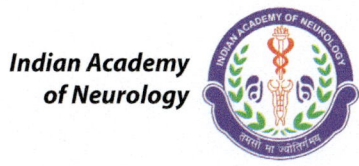

Indian Academy of Neurology

Advances in Stroke

Editor-in-Chief
Debashish Chowdhury
DTCD MD(Medicine) DM(Neurology) FIAN FRCP(Edinburgh)
Commonwealth Fellow in Stroke Medicine(Edinburgh)
Director–Professor and Head
Department of Neurology
GB Pant Institute of Postgraduate Medical Education and Research
New Delhi, India

Editors

PN Sylaja MD(Medicine)
DM(Neurology) FRCP(Edinburgh)
Professor
In-Charge, Comprehensive Stroke Care Program
Sree Chitra Tirunal Institute for Medical Sciences and Technology
Thiruvananthapuram, Kerala, India

VG Pradeep Kumar
MD(Medicine) DM(Neurology) DNB(Neurology)
Senior Consultant
Deputy Chief in Neurology
Stroke Programme
Medical Director
Baby Memorial Hospital
Kozhikode, Kerala, India

Arvind Sharma MD DM RPNI
Head
Department of Neurology
Zydus Hospital
Assistant Professor
SVP Medical College
Ahmedabad, Gujarat, India

Foreword
Subhash Kaul

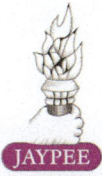

JAYPEE BROTHERS MEDICAL PUBLISHERS
The Health Sciences Publisher
New Delhi | London

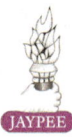 **Jaypee Brothers Medical Publishers (P) Ltd**

Headquarters
EMCA House
23/23-B, Ansari Road, Daryaganj
New Delhi 110 002, India
Landline: +91-11-23272143, +91-11-23272703
+91-11-23282021, +91-11-23245672
E-mail: jaypee@jaypeebrothers.com

Corporate Office
Jaypee Brothers Medical Publishers (P) Ltd.
4838/24, Ansari Road, Daryaganj
New Delhi 110 002, India
Phone: +91-11-43574357
Fax: +91-11-43574314
E-mail: jaypee@jaypeebrothers.com

Overseas Office
JP Medical Ltd.
83, Victoria Street, London
SW1H 0HW (UK)
Phone: +44-20 3170 8910
Fax: +44(0)20 3008 6180
E-mail: info@jpmedpub.com

Website: www.jaypeebrothers.com
Website: www.jaypeedigital.com

© 2025, Jaypee Brothers Medical Publishers

The views and opinions expressed in this book are solely those of the original contributor(s)/author(s) and do not necessarily represent those of editor(s) or publisher of the book.

All rights reserved. No part of this publication may be reproduced, stored or transmitted in any form or by any means, electronic, mechanical, photocopying, recording or otherwise, without the prior permission in writing of the publishers.

All brand names and product names used in this book are trade names, service marks, trademarks or registered trademarks of their respective owners. The publisher is not associated with any product or vendor mentioned in this book.

Medical knowledge and practice change constantly. This book is designed to provide accurate, authoritative information about the subject matter in question. However, readers are advised to check the most current information available on procedures included and check information from the manufacturer of each product to be administered, to verify the recommended dose, formula, method and duration of administration, adverse effects and contraindications. It is the responsibility of the practitioner to take all appropriate safety precautions. Neither the publisher nor the author(s)/editor(s) assume any liability for any injury and/or damage to persons or property arising from or related to use of material in this book.

This book is sold on the understanding that the publisher is not engaged in providing professional medical services. If such advice or services are required, the services of a competent medical professional should be sought.

Every effort has been made where necessary to contact holders of copyright to obtain permission to reproduce copyright material. If any have been inadvertently overlooked, the publisher will be pleased to make the necessary arrangements at the first opportunity.

Inquiries for bulk sales may be solicited at: jaypee@jaypeebrothers.com

IAN Advances in Stroke / Debashish Chowdhury, PN Sylaja, VG Pradeep Kumar, Arvind Sharma

First Edition: 2025
ISBN: 978-93-6616-535-6
Printed in India

Indian Academy of Neurology

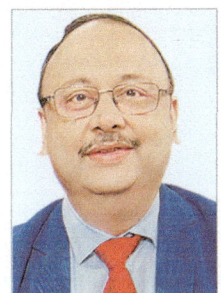

PRESIDENT
Debashish Chowdhury
New Delhi, India

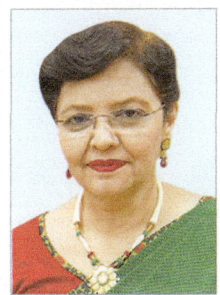

PRESIDENT-ELECT
Sangeeta Ravat
Mumbai, Maharashtra, India

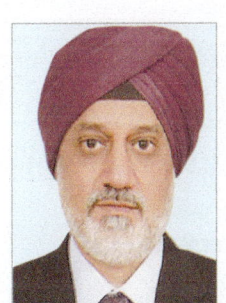

IMMEDIATE PAST PRESIDENT
Gagandeep Singh
Ludhiana, Punjab, India

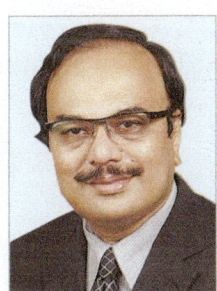

PAST PRESIDENT
Nirmal Surya
Mumbai, Maharashtra, India

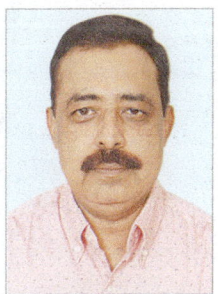

TREASURER
Achal Srivastava
New Delhi, India

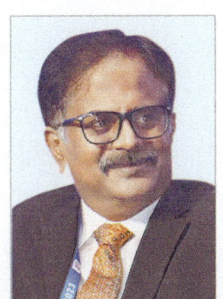

SECRETARY
U Meenakshisundaram
Chennai, Tamil Nadu, India

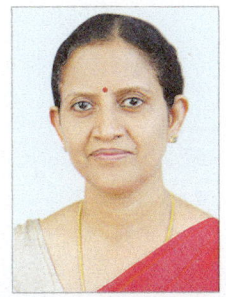

EDITOR, ANNALS OF IAN
PN Sylaja
Thiruvananthapuram, Kerala, India

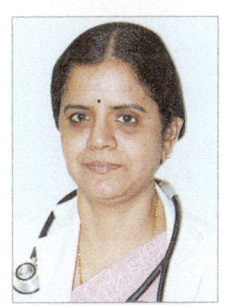

CME CONVENER
Sita Jayalakshmi
Hyderabad, Telangana, India

Executive Members

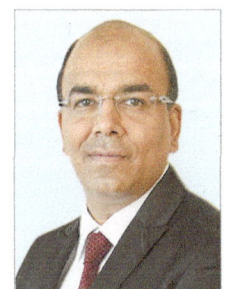

Arvind Sharma
Ahmedabad, Gujarat, India

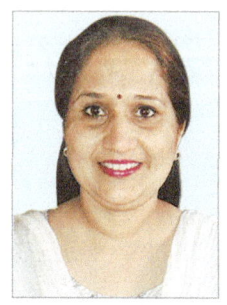

Bhawna Sharma
Jaipur, Rajasthan, India

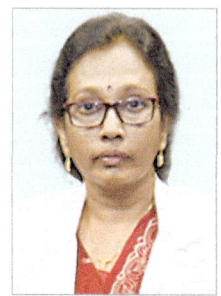

Atchayaram Nalini
Bengaluru, Karnataka, India

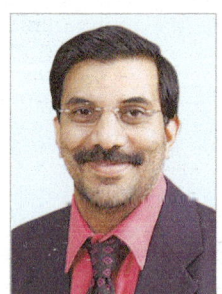

JOINT TREASURER
Pradeep VG
Kozhikode, Kerala, India

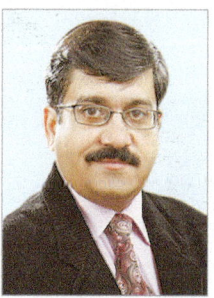

JOINT SECRETARY
Sumit Singh
Gurugram, Haryana, India

Contributors

Col Aneesh Mohimen
MD(Radiodiagnosis)
DM(Neuroradiology)
Professor (Radiodiagnosis) and
Interventional Radiology
Army Hospital (Research and
Referral)
Dhaula Kuan, New Delhi, India

Arun Kathuveetil DNB(Internal
Medicine) DM(Neurology) PDF in
Stroke
Clinical and Research Fellow
Calgary Stroke Program
University of Calgary
Calgary, Alberta, Canada

Arvind Sharma MD DM RPNI
Head
Department of Neurology
Zydus Hospital
Assistant Professor
SVP Medical College
Ahmedabad, Gujarat, India

Ashutosh Mahapatra MD
Assistant Professor
Department of Neurology and
Neurosurgery
Cleveland Clinic Foundation
Lerner College of Medicine
Cleveland, Ohio, USA

Ayush Agarwal DM(Neurology)
Assistant Professor
Department of Neurology
All India Institute of Medical
Sciences
New Delhi, India

Baikuntha Panigrahi
DM(Neurology)
Senior Resident
Department of Neurology
All India Institute of Medical
Sciences
New Delhi, India

Biplab Das MD(Medicine)
DM(Neurology) FINR
Director Neurology and
Neurointervention
Narayana Superspeciality
Hospital
Gurugram, Haryana, India

Debjyoti Dhar DM(Neurology)
Senior Resident
Department of Neurology
National Institute of Mental
Health and Neurosciences
(NIMHANS)
Bengaluru, Karnataka, India

Debsiash Hota MD(Medicine)
DM(Neurology)
Stroke and Neurointervention
Fellow
Consultant Interventional
Neurologist
Narayana Superspeciality
Hospital
Gurugram, Haryana, India

**Diego Antonio Gutierrez
Vasquez** MD
Neurologist
Department of Neurology
School of Medicine, Pontifical
Catholic University of Chile
Santiago, Chile

Dileep R Yavagal MD FSVIN
FAHA FAAN
Professor
Department of Clinical
Neurology and Neurosurgery
Director of Interventional
Neurology
Department of Neurology and
Neurosurgery
University of Miami Miller
School of Medicine and
Jackson Memorial Hospital
Miami, Florida, USA

Girish Baburao Kulkarni
MD(Internal Medicine)
DM(Neurology)
Professor
Department of Neurology
National Institute of Mental
Health and Neurosciences
(NIMHANS)
Bengaluru, Karnataka, India

Kamalesh Chakravarty MD DM
Associate Professor
Department of Neurology
PGIMER
Chandigarh, India

Kameshwar Prasad MD DM
MMSc
Emeritus Professor of
Neurology
AIIMS
New Delhi, India
Dean (Research)
Clinical Research Division
Fortis CSR Foundation
New Delhi, India

MM Samim DM(Neurology)
Senior Resident
Department of Neurology
National Institute of Mental
Health and Neurosciences
(NIMHANS)
Bengaluru, Karnataka, India

Mohan Leslie Noone MD DM
Senior Consultant Neurologist
Baby Memorial Hospital
Kozhikode, Kerala, India

Pallav Bhatter MD(Radio-diagnosis) DNB
Associate Consultant
Neurointervention Surgery
Paras Hospital
Gurugram, Haryana, India

Rajeeb Kumar Mishra MD DESA DM(Neuroanesthesiology and Critical Care)
Consultant, Department of Neuroanesthesia and Neurocritical Care
National Institute of Mental Health and Neurosciences (NIMHANS)
Bengaluru, Karnataka, India
Clinical Fellow
Division of Neurology
National University Hospital
Singapore

Rajesh Kumar Singh MD DM
Additional Professor
Department of Neurology
AIIMS
New Delhi, India

Rajsrinivas Parthasarathy
MRCP CCT(UK, Neurology)
Senior Consultant
Neurointervention Surgery
Paras Hospital
Gurugram, Haryana, India

Sanjith Aaron MD DM(Neurology)
Professor
Department of Neurology
Christian Medical College Hospital Vellore
Vellore, Tamil Nadu, India

Simerpreet S Bal MD DM FRCPC(Neurology)
Clinical Associate Professor
Department of Clinical Neurosciences
University of Calgary
Calgary, Alberta, Canada

Somalin Satapathy
DNB(Anesthesiology)
Critical Care Medicine
Resident
Sir Ganga Ram Hospital
New Delhi, India

Sucharita Ray MD DM PDF FCSC-E
Associate Professor
Department of Neurology
PGIMER
Chandigarh, India

TA Sangeeth DM(Neurology)
Senior Resident
Department of Neurology
National Institute of Mental
Health and Neurosciences
(NIMHANS)
Bengaluru, Karnataka, India

Vijay K Sharma MD FRCP RPNI
Associate Professor
Yong Loo Lin School of Medicine
National University of Singapore
Singapore

Vipul Gupta MD(Radio-diagnosis)
Group Director and Head
Neurointervention Surgery
Paras Hospital
Gurugram, Haryana, India

Foreword

Two important advances in stroke care began in the last decade of the last millennium: The advent of intravenous thrombolysis in ischemic stroke and validation of stroke units for optimum care. Being a fellow at the University of Maryland around that time, I was fortunate to witness these developments from close quarters and subsequently follow the constantly improving and therapeutically important ongoing advances in stroke medicine. There is no doubt that it is crucial for neurologists to stay updated in latest advances to save the patients from preventable disability and death. I compliment the Indian Academy of Neurology in deciding to bring out this book on the recent *Advances in Stroke* and to entrust this responsibility to Drs PN Sylaja, Arvind Sharma, and VG Pradeep Kumar, all eminent stroke specialists and leaders in the field. They have very meticulously chosen the internationally recognized authors of Indian origin having impeccable academic credentials to contribute chapters of high clinical relevance in stroke care. The topics range from advances in stroke imaging, brain hemorrhage, and brain infarcts to the most topical chapter on the role of artificial intelligence in stroke. I have no doubt that all neurology residents and consultants will enjoy reading this book and will also get latest insights and research curiosity to not only improve care of their patients, but also contribute to stroke research.

Subhash Kaul MD DM
Past President, IAN and ISA
Senior Consultant Neurologist
Department of Neurology
Krishna Institute of Medical Sciences
Secunderabad Telangana, India

Message from Editor-in-Chief

Dear Readers,

The Indian Academy of Neurology (IAN) has been at the forefront of neurology education and has a rich history of publications which rank high in terms of academic and scientific content. As President, it has been my pleasure to team up with my Executive Committee members, who are experts in various neurological subspecialties and high-quality and prolific authors with an impressive track record of publications, as editors and bring out a series of books which continue to hold high the tradition of IAN in terms of high-impact scientific content.

As Chief Editor of IAN "*Advances in Stroke*", it is my pleasure to bring to you a book which sets the bar high for content—accurate, updated, and relevant—and at the same time presents it in a reader-friendly manner, which makes the book an ideal companion for everyone interested in the subject. I thank my colleagues and editors of this book, *Dr PN Sylaja, Dr VG Pradeep Kumar and Dr Arvind Sharma*, for the shared vision of high-quality, focused content as well as excellent support rendered during the making of this book.

This has been our collective effort, and we sincerely hope that each of you will like reading this book as much as we loved bringing this out.

Debashish Chowdhury

Preface

Stroke is a leading cause of mortality and disability in both developed and developing countries. Recently, the scientific and technological advances of the last few decades have drastically changed the landscape of acute stroke diagnosis and management. For a long time, stroke management was clouded by a sense of therapeutic nihilism, as clinicians felt helpless in the face of such a devastating condition. However, with the advent of intravenous thrombolysis in the 1990s, the landscape of stroke care began to change dramatically. With the extended window for intravenous thrombolysis and endovascular thrombectomy, we have opportunities to treat more patients acutely. This pivotal advancement ushered in a new era of stroke research, transforming the field from one of stagnation to making significant strides in understanding the causes, progression, and treatment of stroke. Today, the global burden of stroke calls for constant innovation, as the challenge lies not only in acute management but also in preventing recurrent events and minimizing long-term disability.

This book is a timely compilation of the latest advances in stroke care. It brings together insights from globally renowned experts in the field, addressing a wide range of topics, including cutting-edge imaging techniques and artificial intelligence applications to new therapeutic approaches like endovascular thrombectomy and the management of intracerebral hemorrhage.

Comprising 11 chapters, this book offers a comprehensive overview of the developments that are reshaping stroke care. We believe that this volume will serve as a resource for clinicians, providing nuanced insights that will enhance diagnosis, treatment, and patient care in patients with stroke.

Bringing together this compendium on recent advances in stroke management has been an immensely rewarding endeavor, and we are deeply grateful to all those who contributed to its success. We would like to extend our sincere thanks to the Indian Academy of Neurology (IAN) for providing us with the opportunity to lead this important project.

This volume would not have been possible without the unwavering dedication and expertise of the contributing authors, each of whom has shared invaluable insights in their respective fields. We are grateful to each one of them. Their collective expertise has enriched this book, making it a valuable resource for clinicians.

We would also like to express our deep appreciation to the publication team at Jaypee Brothers Medical Publishers, particularly Ms Chetna Malhotra (Senior Director—Professional Publishing, Marketing and Business Development) and Ms Nedup Bhutia Pillai (Assistant Manager—Print Publishing), for their unwavering support and diligence in bringing this book to life. Their meticulous work has transformed a vision into reality.

Lastly, we are indebted to Dr Debashish Chowdhury for his constant guidance throughout this project, helping shape the book into a comprehensive and relevant resource for the medical community.

The IAN has once again spearheaded an outstanding series, contributing to the ongoing evolution of stroke management.

PN Sylaja
VG Pradeep Kumar
Aravind Sharma

Contents

CHAPTER 1: **Recent Advances of Transcranial Doppler in Acute Stroke**   1
Arvind Sharma, Rajeeb Kumar Mishra, Vijay K Sharma

CHAPTER 2: **Recent Advances in the Management of Spontaneous Intracerebral Hemorrhage**   12
Baikuntha Panigrahi, Ayush Agarwal

CHAPTER 3: **Advances in Intravenous Thrombolysis**   26
Rajesh Kumar Singh, Kameshwar Prasad

CHAPTER 4: **Artificial Intelligence in Acute Stroke Management**   40
Mohan Leslie Noone

CHAPTER 5: **Expanding Indications in Acute Ischemic Stroke Reperfusion and Endovascular Therapy**   47
Ashutosh Mahapatra, Dileep R Yavagal

CHAPTER 6: **Management of Direct-acting Oral Anticoagulant–Associated Intracerebral Hemorrhage**   61
Sucharita Ray, Kamalesh Chakravarty

CHAPTER 7: **Aortic Arch Atheroma—Underdiagnosed Stroke Mechanism: Diagnosis and Management**   70
Simerpreet S Bal, Arun Kathuveetil, Diego Antonio Gutierrez Vasquez

CHAPTER 8: **Recent Advances in the Management of Cerebral Venous Thrombosis**   83
Debjyoti Dhar, TA Sangeeth, MM Samim, Sanjith Aaron, Girish Baburao Kulkarni

CHAPTER 9: **Misinterpretations in Vessel Wall Magnetic Resonance Imaging: Essential Insights**   96
Pallav Bhatter, Rajsrinivas Parthasarathy, Vipul Gupta

CHAPTER 10:   **Beyond Antithrombotic in Secondary Prevention of Stroke**   111
Debsiash Hota, Biplab Das, Somalin Satapathy

CHAPTER 11:   **Recent Advances in Imaging of Acute Ischemic Stroke**   123
Aneesh Mohimen

Index   143

CHAPTER 1

Recent Advances of Transcranial Doppler in Acute Stroke

Arvind Sharma, Rajeeb Kumar Mishra, Vijay K Sharma

ABSTRACT

Transcranial Doppler (TCD) ultrasonography remains the only noninvasive imaging modality that allows a reliable evaluation of cerebral hemodynamics in the major arteries of the circle of Willis. TCD is relatively cheaper and bedside tool that enables extended continuous monitoring of the changes in blood flow patterns in real-time, especially in response to intravenous thrombolysis and endovascular procedures. While continuous ultrasound exposure of the offending blood clot enhances the chances of recanalization induced by intravenous thrombolytic agent, the real-time information provided by TCD may help in determining the optimal timing of other neuroimaging studies as well as additional therapeutic interventions. Furthermore, advanced applications of TCD help in understanding the stroke mechanism as well as taking various therapeutic decisions for secondary stroke prevention. In this chapter, we provide various diagnostic, therapeutic, as well as prognostic applications of TCD in patients with acute ischemic stroke.

Keywords: Transcranial Doppler, Acute ischemic stroke, Sonothrombolysis, Cerebral hemodynamics.

■ INTRODUCTION

Rapid developments in neurovascular imaging during past two decades have led to revolutionizing the development of current reperfusion strategies. Transcranial Doppler (TCD) is a noninvasive, portable, and reliable tool for a rapid detection of the offending intracranial arterial occlusion in acute ischemic stroke.[1] In addition, continuous TCD monitoring in patients with large artery occlusion helps in monitoring the response to intravenous thrombolysis, safely enhancing the effects of thrombolysis (sonothrombolysis), in addition to selecting patients for endovascular therapy (EVT). Finally, advanced applications of TCD may also help in establishing the cause of stroke as well as facilitating various interventions for secondary stroke prevention.[2] This chapter provides an overview of the current role of TCD in the management of acute ischemic stroke.

■ TRANSCRANIAL DOPPLER AS COMPARED TO OTHER VASCULAR IMAGING MODALITIES

Various neuroimaging modalities may provide crucial information about the status of arterial occlusion, collaterals, the extent, and severity of ischemia in patients with acute ischemic stroke. Computerized tomographic angiography (CTA) and magnetic resonance angiography (MRA) are the two imaging modalities commonly employed to assess arterial patency in acute stroke. However, both imaging methods provide only the anatomical "snap shot" about the presence of an intracranial arterial occlusion at the time of imaging, instead of the "ever-changing or dynamic" status of the arterial patency in acute ischemic stroke. On the other hand, TCD permits longitudinal and extended monitoring of the intracranial arterial occlusion, its downstream hemodynamic effects, as well the information about recanalization, if any, in response to various recanalization strategies employed in acute ischemic stroke patients. However, CT and MRI score over TCD by providing additional information about the location and extent of the cerebral parenchymal damage. We wish to reiterate that the hemodynamic information provided by TCD is not a duplication of the findings on CT/CTA or MRI/MRA. Instead, TCD provides complementary information (which is physiological) to the anatomical imaging and helps the clinician to understand the stroke process better.[3]

TRANSCRANIAL DOPPLER IN HYPERACUTE ISCHEMIC STROKE: DIAGNOSTIC

Although most secondary and tertiary centers perform urgent CT/CTA or MRI/MRA upon arrival of an acute ischemic stroke to the emergency room, TCD still finds a useful role. While TCD may be the primary imaging modality at primary medical centers or peripheral hospitals, it may be used to confirm the presence of intracranial arterial occlusion and/or monitor the arterial patency in response to recanalization therapies (especially intravenous thrombolysis). Chernyshev et al. in 2005 developed a fast-track TCD insonation protocol for patients with acute ischemic stroke, which could be completed within minutes by the treating neurologist, sonographer, or stroke nurse, who possess the clinical knowledge about the patient.[4] Accordingly, TCD is started on the suspected side to evaluate the presumed occluded intracranial artery. In patients who have already undergone CTA/MRA upon arrival to the emergency room, sonographer can find the occluded intracranial artery, measure the distance of occlusion site from skin surface on the scan, and obtain the residual TCD flow signals. TCD has a high yield in hyperacute ischemic stroke patients and may demonstrate an intracranial arterial occlusion in up to 90% of patients who are eligible for thrombolytic therapy, especially if the National Institute of Health Stroke Scale (NIHSS) is 10 points or more. Interestingly, a normal TCD examination in hyperacute ischemic stroke patients has >96% specificity in excluding an arterial occlusion. Overall, TCD carries excellent accuracy parameters when compared to CTA or MRA in patients presenting with acute ischemic stroke.[5,6]

COLLATERALS IMAGING WITH TRANSCRANIAL DOPPLER

In addition to the detection of intracranial occlusion in acute stroke patients, TCD may help in the assessment of collateral blood flow, widely believed to prolong the ischemic penumbra and improving functional outcomes.[7] One of the most important collaterals is the anterior cross-filling via anterior communicating artery (Acomm) in patients with acute occlusive disease of internal carotid artery (ICA). This is observed as elevated flow velocities in anterior cerebral artery (ACA) on side contralateral to the ICA occlusion. Accordingly, the A1 ACA on the affected side shows reversed flow. Since a large amount of blood flows through the ACom, TCD usually shows stenotic-like flow (even with a musical bruit in some cases) at depths of 72–78 mm directed away from the donor side. Middle cerebral artery (MCA) on the recipient side may show blunted Doppler spectra.

Posterior communication artery (PComm) serves as another collateral pathway to perfuse the MCA on the side of ICA occlusive disease. In such cases, a low-resistance flow directed mostly toward the TCD probe is observed at depths of 58–68 mm, located posterior to ICA bifurcation.[7]

Another common observation noted in patients with acute intracranial arterial occlusion is flow diversion. Since the blood flow in major intracranial arteries is all about the presence of branches. As a result, once a main arterial branch is occluded, blood tends to go into the adjacent branch (flow diversion), common examples include flow diversion to ipsilateral ACA in patients with M1 MCA occlusion, where MCA mean flow velocity (MFV) will be lower than ipsilateral ACA, in addition to the higher resistance in the MCA **(Fig. 1)** and flow diversion into M2 MCA when other M2 MCA occludes.[7]

■ TRANSCRANIAL DOPPLER IN HYPERACUTE ISCHEMIC STROKE: MONITORING

In acute ischemic stroke, especially due to large vessel occlusion (LVO), achieving arterial recanalization is considered the key for ensuring better functional outcomes.[8] Currently, most stroke centers initiate intravenous thrombolysis with tissue plasminogen activator (IV-tPA) in eligible acute

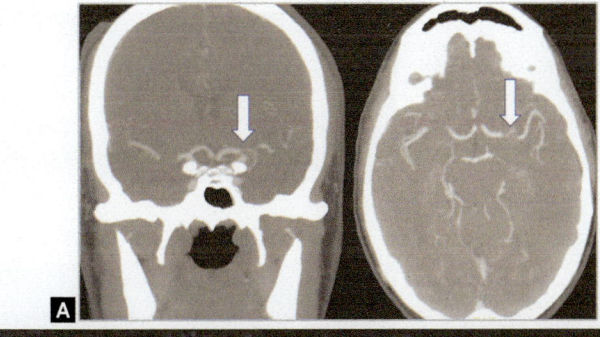

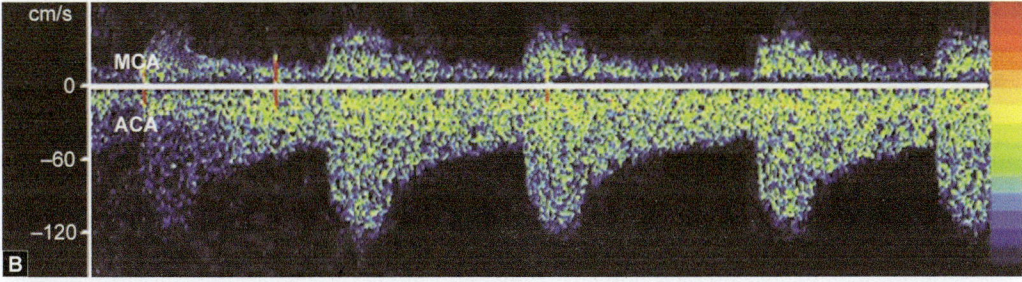

FIGS. 1A AND B: TCD findings in acute left middle cerebral artery occlusion. This 64-year-old man presented with sudden onset of right-sided weakness and inability to speak for about 2 hours. National Institute of Health Stroke Scale (NIHSS) was 14 points. (A) Shows a filling defect in proximal left middle cerebral artery (MCA) in coronal and axial planes on CT angiography. Bedside TCD (B) shows low flow velocities (with high resistance pattern) in the MCA, consistent with an acute partial occlusion. Note the flow velocities in ipsilateral ACA are higher than the MCA (with lower resistance), representing flow diversion.

(ACA: anterior cerebral artery; TCD: transcranial Doppler)

stroke and immediately shift them for EVT if there is an LVO.

For patients undergoing EVT, contrast angiography provides real-time information about the status of arterial patency; this information is often missing in patients who are treated with only IV-tPA due to various patient-specific reasons. In such cases, TCD monitoring plays an important role by demonstrating the timing and extent of arterial recanalization induced by IV-tPA **(Fig. 2)**. Such information is specifically relevant in patients who show clinical improvement, clinical deterioration following improvement as well as fluctuating neurological examination.[9] In addition, the new TCD findings may even prompt the stroke neurologist to even reconsider EVT in some cases.

Interestingly, when compared to contrast angiography, TCD is highly sensitivite and specific (91% and 93%, respectively) for complete occlusion versus complete recanalization of MCA in acute ischemic stroke patients treated with IV-tPA. The Thrombolysis in Brain Ischemia (TIBI) flow grading system, developed by Demchuk et al., is used for objective evaluation of the residual flow in occluded intracranial arteries as well as to monitor the recanalization in real-time, if any.[10] TIBI flow grades correlate with stroke severity and mortality, in addition

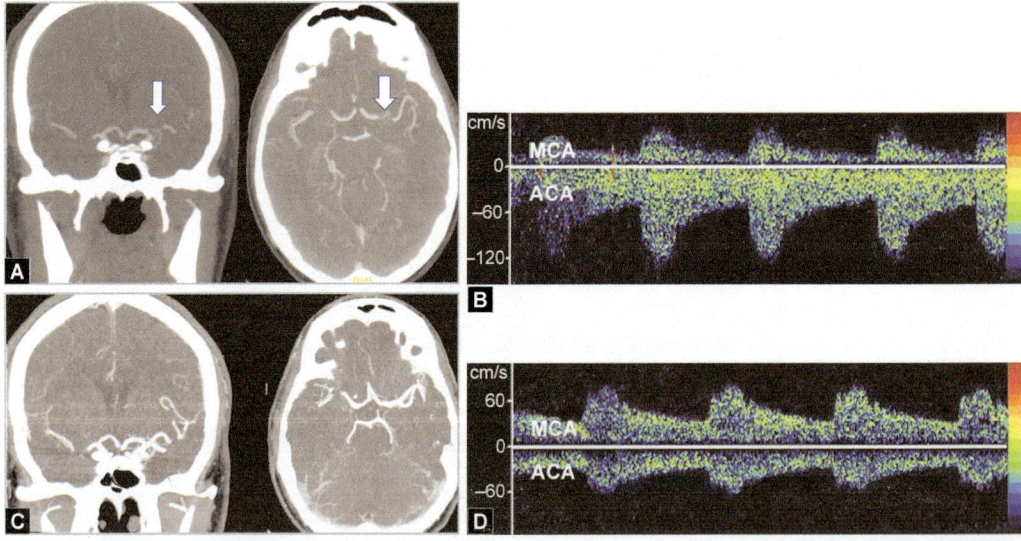

FIGS. 2A TO D: Serial TCD findings in a patient with acute left middle cerebral artery occlusion treated with intravenous thrombolysis (same patient in Fig. 1). This 64-year-old man presented with sudden onset of right-sided weakness and inability to speak for about 2 hours. National Institute of Health Stroke Scale (NIHSS) was 14 points. (A) Shows a filling defect in proximal left middle cerebral artery (MCA) in coronal and axial planes on CT angiography. Bedside TCD (B) shows low flow velocities (with high resistance pattern) in the MCA, consistent with an acute partial occlusion. Note the flow velocities in ipsilateral ACA are higher than the MCA (with lower resistance), representing flow diversion. Intravenous thrombolysis with tissue plasminogen activator (IV-tPA) was initiated at 135 minutes from symptom-onset and continuous TCD monitoring was performed. He showed rapid neurological recovery within 20 minutes of IV-tPA bolus. CT angiography performed at 45 minutes after IV-tPA bolus (C) shows complete recanalization of left MCA. Corresponding TCD findings (normalization of flow velocities and resistance in MCA and resolution of flow diversion to ipsilateral ACA) are presented in (D).

(ACA: anterior cerebral artery; TCD: transcranial Doppler)

to the likelihood of recanalization and clinical improvement. Broadly, TIBI grades 2–3 represent partial, and TIBI grades 4–5 indicate complete recanalization.

A recent multicenter, prospective observational cohort study of 480 patients evaluated the feasibility of continuous TCD monitoring in thrombolysed acute stroke patients and to determine whether early (within 1-hour from IV-tPA-bolus) complete or partial recanalization is associated with better outcomes in patients with LVO.[11] The study outcomes were dramatic clinical recovery (DCR) within first 24 hours from IV-tPA-bolus, mortality at 3 months, in addition to favorable functional outcome (FFO) and functional independence (FI) defined as modified Rankin Scale (mRS) scores of 0–1 and 0–2, respectively. The study reported that early recanalization (53%) was significantly associated with higher rates of DCR at 2 hours (54% vs. 10%) and 24 hours (63% vs. 22%), 3 months FFO (67% vs. 28%), and FI (81% vs. 39%). Interestingly, 3-month mortality rates (6% vs. 17%) were significantly lower in the early recanalization group. After adjusting for potential confounders, early recanalization was independently associated with higher odds of 3-month FFO [odds ratio (OR) 6.19; 95% confidence interval (CI) 3.88–9.88] and lower likelihood of 3-month mortality (OR 0.34; 95% CI 0.17–0.67).[11]

■ THERAPEUTIC ROLE OF TRANSCRANIAL DOPPLER: SONOTHROMBOLYSIS

The mainstay of the treatment during hyperacute ischemic stroke treatment is achieving recanalization of the occluded intracranial artery. However, the recanalization rates in thrombolysed acute ischemic stroke patients are unacceptably low. del Zoppo et al. showed that only 26% of intracranial occlusions lyse partially or completely after 1 hour of intravenous duteplase infusion.[12] Similarly, low rates of arterial recanalization have been observed in studies that used IV-tPA, especially in the occlusions of proximal intracranial arteries.[13,14]

Despite receiving timely thrombolysis, almost half of the patients remain moderately or severely disabled. One important reason for this poor rate of recovery is slow and incomplete thrombolysis. Thus, the quest for improving recanalization rates continued, especially using transcranial ultrasound exposure during IV-tPA infusion. Encouraging findings were observed during various in vitro experiments in the form of significantly improved and faster dissolution of the blood clots by tPA, when exposed to continuous exposure to ultrasound of lower frequency (kHz) range.[15-18] Even the 2-MHz transducer in the commercially available diagnostic TCD machines transmits sufficient amount of ultrasound energy to the intracranial vessels, to enhance the activity of IV-tPA. This was seen in the pivotal CLOTBUST randomized clinical trial. This trial randomly assigned (1:1) 126 patients to continuous TCD (2-MHz) monitoring or placebo in addition to IV-tPA. Complete recanalization or DCR within 2 hours after IV-tPA bolus was noted in 49% in the TCD group as compared to only 30% in the control group ($p = 0.03$).[19] Interestingly, there was no increase in symptomatic intracerebral hemorrhage (SICH).

Subsequently, many meta-analyses showed the safety and efficacy of sonothrombolysis, with a nearly threefold increased likelihood of complete recanalization and twofold higher likelihood of FI at 3 months.[20]

Augmenting Sonothrombolysis: Ultrasound Contrast Agents

Commercially available ultrasound contrast agents enhance the quality of images due to improved reflection strength. When exposed to the pulsed-wave ultrasound, these microbubbles/microspheres undergo transient oscillations (compression and expansion) in size, leading to their disruption, transmitting mechanical energy momentum, which helps in mechanical clot dissolution. This phenomenon was evaluated in many studies on thrombolysed acute ischemic stroke patients.

An initial observational study compared 103 consecutive acute ischemic stroke patients with occluded MCA who received either IV-tPA alone, IV-tPA plus continuous TCD monitoring, or IV-tPA, TCD, and ultrasound contrast (Levovist) injections. Complete recanalization at 2 hours was 54.5% in the Levovist/TCD/tPA group, 40.8% in the ultrasound/tPA group, and 23.9% in the tPA-alone group. Importantly, neurological improvement was significantly better in the Levovist/TCD/tPA group.[21] However, the early generation microbubbles were air-filled, making them "bubble-up" in saline and rise up in the intravenous solutions, making continuous infusion difficult. Furthermore, their bigger size and weak shells reduced their presence time in systemic circulation. This led to a feasibility and safety trial by using novel and more stable lipid coated microspheres containing an inert gas (perflutren).[22] Although improved rates of arterial recanalization were observed but the trial was stopped prematurely due to commercial reasons. This was followed by the transcranial ultrasound in clinical sonolysis (TUCSON) trial which was a dose-escalation trial designed to determine the optimal dose of the more stable MRX-801 nanobubble platform for enhancing the arterial recanalization when acute ischemic stroke patients underwent continuous TCD monitoring during IV-tPA infusion.[22] Improved recanalization rates were observed among the patients treated during first-dose tier. However, two patients in the second dose-tier developed SICH (deemed related to uncontrolled blood pressure), leading to the withdrawal of commercial funding and unfortunate premature closure of the trial.

Since TCD monitoring capabilities were not available widely, attempts were made to develop hands-free headsets that were made of multiple transducer crystals oriented in various directions to deliver 2-MHz continuous ultrasound to all the main arteries of the circle of Willis (both anterior and posterior circulation). The headset did not have any visual or audio output and could be easily mounted (even by medical personnel not expert in TCD) on the head of the patients. This hands-free headset was evaluated in a multinational randomized clinical trial (CLOTBUSTER) in acute ischemic stroke patients receiving IV-tPA infusion.[23] Using 1:1 central randomization (continuous 2-MHz ultrasound exposure or sham treatment). Although the trial showed the feasibility and safety of using hands-free ultrasound device, it was stopped prematurely due to futility. One possible reason for the observed results from this trial was the announcement of highly encouraging results of MR-CLEAN trial, which affected the rate and quality of patient recruitment into the CLOTBUSTER trial.[24]

ROLE OF TRANSCRANIAL DOPPLER IN THE ERA OF MECHANICAL THROMBECTOMY

Mechanical thrombectomy, also called endovascular thrombectomy (EVT), employs a device passed intra-arterially for physical removal of clots in acute ischemic stroke patients with LVO. A meta-analysis of the individual patient database from five large randomized clinical trials of acute ischemic stroke due to LVO in anterior circulation ($n = 1287$) showed that EVT significantly reduced disability at 90 days compared with a control (adjusted cOR 2.49; 95% CI 1.76–3.53).[25]

Using the database of our CLOTBUST-PRO registry,[11] we examined the clinical utility and prognostic value of TCD flow findings by assessing the MFV ratio, comparing the reciprocal ratios of MCAs bilaterally [affected MCA-to-contralateral MCA MFV (aMCA/cMCA MFV ratio)].[26] Of the total of 222 patients with LVO on CTA, 88 patients had M1 MCA occlusions with their baseline mean NIHSS score of 16 points, and a 24-hour mean NIHSS score of 10 points. We found that an aMCA/cMCA MFV ratio of <0.6 had a sensitivity of 99%, specificity of 16%, positive predictive value (PV) of 60%, and negative PV of 94% for identifying M1 MCA, terminal ICA, or tandem ICA/MCA acute occlusion. TIBI grade ≥1 compared to grade 0 showed a sensitivity of 17.1%, specificity of 86.9%, positive PV of 62%, and negative PV of 46% for identifying LVO. Our findings demonstrate a possible potential for TCD as a screening tool for IV thrombolysis as well as EVT protocols.

ROLE OF TRANSCRANIAL DOPPLER IN PATIENT SELECTION FOR EARLY INTERVENTIONS FOR STROKE PREVENTION

Hyperacute treatment with IV thrombolysis and/or EVT holds the key for limiting the morbidity, mortality, as well as ensuring a FFO in acute ischemic stroke patients. However, secondary stroke prevention holds an equally important position in acute ischemic stroke patients. While the use of appropriate antithrombotic therapy and optimal control of various vascular risk are universally recommended, efforts are made to detect certain high-risk and potentially treatable conditions. We will discuss two specific conditions where TCD plays an important role, namely detection of spontaneous emboli in patients with large artery atherosclerosis and right-to-left shunt in patients with paradoxical embolism.

Transcranial Doppler Emboli Detection

Microembolic signals (MES) appear as transient ultrasound signals with high intensity within the TCD spectra. The only diagnostic modality that can detect MES is ultrasound since MES have different acoustic properties compared to the flowing blood **(Fig. 3)**.

Typical characteristics of MES include their random appearance within the cardiac cycle and the characteristic "chirp", "click", or "whistle" sound.

Detection of MES is particularly important when the cerebral ischemic symptoms are due to embolism from an unstable atherosclerotic plaque in a major cervical or intracranial artery, aortic arch atheroma, or cardioembolic source. TCD MES monitoring was used as a surrogate marker to evaluate the effectiveness of medical treatment in the CARESS trial (Clopidogrel and Aspirin for Reduction of Emboli in Symptomatic Carotid Stenosis), which showed that the combination of clopidogrel and aspirin was significantly better than aspirin alone in reducing MES and adverse event in patients with symptomatic carotid artery stenosis.[27] Similar benefits of dual antiplatelet therapy were observed among patients with acute cerebral ischemia due to atherosclerosis of intracranial ICA or proximal MCA.[28] Thus, TCD emboli monitoring could help in selecting the optimal antithrombotic therapy, especially when artery-to-artery embolization is the underlying mechanism of cerebral ischemia.

In a considerable proportion of patients with acute ischemic stroke, the underlying cause is the presence of significant carotid artery stenosis. While most centers plan carotid revascularization procedure within 2-4 weeks of an acute cerebral ischemic event, persistence of MES on TCD monitoring despite optimal medical therapy may be

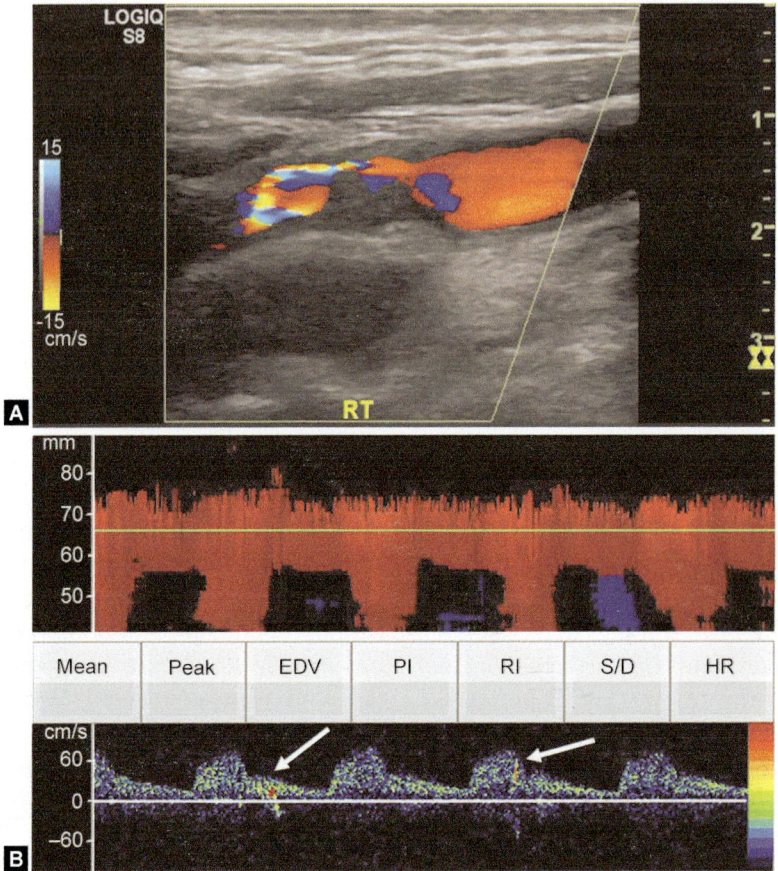

FIGS. 3A AND B: Neurosonological findings in a patient with carotid stenosis. A 68-year-old man presented with sudden onset of left-sided weakness for 6-hour duration. NIHSS was 12-points. CT scan of the brain did not show any bleed. However, hyperdense MCA sign was noted on the right MCA, confirmed by an occluded right proximal MCA on CT angiography. A severe focal stenosis was noted in the proximal cervical internal carotid artery (ICA). Urgently performed mechanical thrombectomy resulted in achieving complete recanalization of the right MCA, accompanied by neurological recovery (NIHSS 3 points). We planned carotid revascularization electively at a later date. CT scan performed on day 2 showed a small infarct in right basal ganglia and no intracerebral hemorrhage was noted. He was started on dual antiplatelet therapy and high-dose statin. However, on day 3, he developed two transient episodes of new weakness on the left face and upper limb. An urgent cervical duplex ultrasonography confirmed a severe focal stenosis of the right proximal ICA (A). Continuous TCD monitoring of right MCA revealed frequent microembolic signals (arrows) for 30 minutes (B). He underwent an uneventful right ICA stenting on day 3 and did not have any recurrence of cerebral ischemic symptoms and achieved complete recovery at 3 months.

(EDV: end-diastolic velocity; HR: heart rate; MCA: middle cerebral artery; NIHSS: National Institute of Health Stroke Scale; PI: pulsatility index; RI: resistance index; S/D: systolic-diastolic ratio; TCD: transcranial Doppler)

used as a criterion for performing an early carotid intervention. Furthermore, TCD can help in further therapeutic decision-making by assessing the downstream intracranial hemodynamic effects of carotid stenosis, identifying additional intracranial stenotic lesions (tandem lesions) as well as evaluating the vasomotor reactivity in the MCA ipsilateral to the stenosis for further risk stratification.[29]

Transcranial Doppler for Right-to-left Shunt Detection

Patent foramen ovale (PFO) is the most common type of right-to-left shunt, with a prevalence of 10–35% among the general population. The reported prevalence is even higher in patients with cryptogenic stroke or transient ischemic attack (TIA) and especially in younger patients without an apparent etiology.[30]

While contrast enhanced transesophageal echocardiography (TEE) is the gold standard for the diagnosis of PFO, it remains a partially invasive procedure due to the involved endoscopy tube. Furthermore, the presence of endoscope tube in the throat limits patients' ability to perform an adequate Valsalva maneuver, limiting the ability of TEE in detecting small and low functional grade PFOs.

Transcranial Doppler serves as an optimal method for detecting the MES in cerebral circulation with high sensitivity and specificity. In addition to the detection of a right-to-left shunt, TCD allows functional grading of the shunt.[31,32] TCD is considered as more sensitive and specific than TEE for RLS detection as well as quantifying its "functional-potential". The test involves injection of agitated contrast mixture (9 mL saline + 1 mL air + few drops of patient's blood) into a large peripheral vein while monitoring an intracranial artery. After injecting the contrast mixture, patient is asked to perform Valsalva maneuver and TCD monitoring is continued for about 25 seconds **(Fig. 4)**. The test can be repeated in multiple body positions to improve the accuracy for grading the shunt severity.[33] It is important to note that TCD does not diagnose the location or type of shunt. However, TCD helps in selecting patients with significant shunts for TEE to determine the anatomical location and feasibility of closure for secondary stroke prevention.

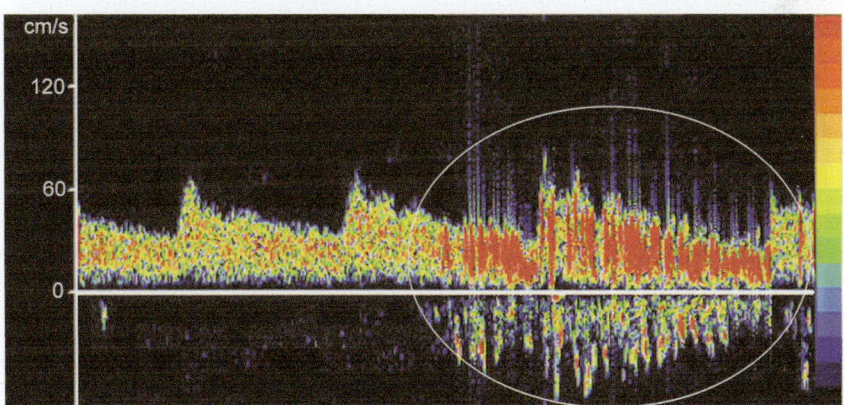

FIG. 4: TCD findings in a patient with acute ischemic stroke due to paradoxical embolism. A 43-year-old woman presented with sudden onset of left-sided weakness for 3 hours. She did not suffer from any cardiovascular risk factor. Her NIHSS upon arrival was 5 points. An urgent CT scan of the brain was unremarkable. However, a filling defect was noted in one of the right distal M2 MCA branch. She was treated with intravenous tissue plasminogen activator. Continuous TCD monitoring resulted in complete recanalization the right M2 MCA, accompanied by complete neurological recovery (NIHSS 0 point at completion of thrombolytic infusion). Later, TCD bubble study showed a large functional grade right-to-left shunt (marked by a curtain of microembolic signals on TCD shown in the figure). Transesophageal echocardiography confirmed the presence of an atrial septal defect as well as patent foramen ovale, which were closed endovascularly. She has remained asymptomatic for past 4 years.

(MCA: middle cerebral artery; NIHSS: National Institute of Health Stroke Scale; TCD: transcranial Doppler)

CONCLUSION

In summary, TCD is an excellent bedside tool during diagnostic workup of hyperacute ischemic stroke patients, and considered as an essential component of modern comprehensive stroke centers. In addition to empowering the treating neurologists to monitor the dynamic changes in cerebral blood flow in thrombolysed acute ischemic stroke, TCD enhances the speed and amount of clot dissolution induced by various fibrinolytic agents. Furthermore, various advanced applications of TCD provide useful information about the underlying mechanisms of neurological fluctuations in patients with acute ischemic stroke, which may help in optimal timing of performing appropriate neuroimaging studies as well as therapeutic decision making during the early phase and preventing stroke recurrence.

REFERENCES

1. Alexandrov AV, Sloan MA, Tegeler CH, Newell DN, Lumsden A, Garami Z, et al.; American Society of Neuroimaging Practice Guidelines Committee. Practice standards for transcranial Doppler (TCD) ultrasound. Part II. Clinical indications and expected outcomes. J Neuroimaging. 2012;22(3):215-24.
2. Sharma VK, Tsivgoulis G, Lao AY, Alexandrov AV. Role of transcranial Doppler ultrasonography in evaluation of patients with cerebrovascular disease. Curr Neurol Neurosci Rep. 2007;7(1):8-20.
3. Yeo LL, Sharma VK. Role of transcranial Doppler ultrasonography in cerebrovascular disease. Recent Pat CNS Drug Discov. 2010;5(1):1-13.
4. Chernyshev OY, Garami Z, Calleja S, Song J, Campbell MS, Noser EA, et al. Yield and accuracy of urgent combined carotid/transcranial ultrasound testing in acute cerebral ischemia. Stroke. 2005;36(1):32-7.
5. Tsivgoulis G, Sharma VK, Lao AY, Malkoff MD, Alexandrov AV. Validation of transcranial Doppler with computed tomography angiography in acute cerebral ischemia. Stroke. 2007;38(4):1245-9.
6. Boddu DB, Sharma VK, Bandaru VC, Jyotsna Y, Padmaja D, Suvarna A, et al. Validation of transcranial Doppler with magnetic resonance angiography in acute cerebral ischemia. J Neuroimaging. 2011;21(2):e34-40.
7. Saqqur M, Khan K, Derksen C, Alexandrov A, Shuaib A. Transcranial Doppler and Transcranial Color Duplex in Defining Collateral Cerebral Blood Flow. J Neuroimaging. 2018;28(5):455-76.
8. Rha JH, Saver JL. The impact of recanalization on ischemic stroke outcome: a meta-analysis. Stroke. 2007;38(3):967-73.
9. Alexandrov AV, Felberg RA, Demchuk AM, Christou I, Burgin WS, Malkoff M, et al. Deterioration following spontaneous improvement: sonographic findings in patients with acutely resolving symptoms of cerebral ischemia. Stroke. 2000;31(4):915-9.
10. Demchuk AM, Burgin WS, Christou I, Felberg RA, Barber PA, Hill MD, et al. Thrombolysis in brain ischemia (TIBI) transcranial Doppler flow grades predict clinical severity, early recovery, and mortality in patients treated with intravenous tissue plasminogen activator. Stroke. 2001;32(1):89-93.
11. Tsivgoulis G, Saqqur M, Sharma VK, Brunser A, Eggers J, Mikulik R, et al.; CLOTBUST-PRO investigators. Timing of Recanalization and Functional Recovery in Acute Ischemic Stroke. J Stroke. 2020;22(1):130-40.
12. del Zoppo GJ, Poeck K, Pessin MS, Wolpert SM, Furlan AJ, Ferbert A, et al. Recombinant tissue plasminogen activator in acute thrombotic and embolic stroke. Ann Neurol. 1992;32(1):78-86.
13. Zangerle A, Kiechl S, Spiegel M, Furtner M, Knoflach M, Werner P, et al. Recanalization after thrombolysis in stroke patients: predictors and prognostic implications. Neurology. 2007;68(1):39-44.
14. Ribo M, Alvarez-Sabín J, Montaner J, Romero F, Delgado P, Rubiera M, et al. Temporal profile of recanalization after intravenous tissue plasminogen activator: selecting patients for rescue reperfusion techniques. Stroke. 2006;37(4):1000-4.
15. Spengos K, Behrens S, Daffertshofer M, Dempfle CE, Hennerici M. Acceleration of thrombolysis

with ultrasound through the cranium in a flow model. Ultrasound Med Biol. 2000;26(5):889-95.
16. Braaten JV, Goss RA, Francis CW. Ultrasound reversibly disaggregates fibrin fibers. Thromb Haemost. 1997;78(3):1063-8.
17. Kondo I, Mizushige K, Ueda T, Masugata H, Ohmori K, Matsuo H. Histological observations and the process of ultrasound contrast agent enhancement of tissue plasminogen activator thrombolysis with ultrasound exposure. Jpn Circ J. 1999;63(6):478-84.
18. Suchkova V, Siddiqi FN, Carstensen EL, Dalecki D, Child S, Francis CW. Enhancement of fibrinolysis with 40-kHz ultrasound. Circulation. 1998;98(10):1030-5.
19. Alexandrov AV, Molina CA, Grotta JC, Garami Z, Ford SR, Alvarez-Sabin J, et al.; CLOTBUST Investigators. Ultrasound-enhanced systemic thrombolysis for acute ischemic stroke. N Engl J Med. 2004;351(21):2170-8.
20. Saqqur M, Tsivgoulis G, Nicoli F, Skoloudik D, Sharma VK, Larrue V, et al. The role of sonolysis and sonothrombolysis in acute ischemic stroke: a systematic review and meta-analysis of randomized controlled trials and case-control studies. J Neuroimaging. 2014;24(3):209-20.
21. Molina CA, Ribo M, Rubiera M, Montaner J, Santamarina E, Delgado-Mederos R, et al. Microbubble administration accelerates clot lysis during continuous 2-MHz ultrasound monitoring in stroke patients treated with intravenous tissue plasminogen activator. Stroke. 2006;37(2):425-9.
22. Alexandrov AV, Mikulik R, Ribo M, Sharma VK, Lao AY, Tsivgoulis G, et al. A pilot randomized clinical safety study of sonothrombolysis augmentation with ultrasound-activated perflutren-lipid microspheres for acute ischemic stroke. Stroke. 2008;39(5):1464-9.
23. Alexandrov AV, Köhrmann M, Soinne L, Tsivgoulis G, Barreto AD, Demchuk AM, et al.; CLOTBUST-ER Trial Investigators. Safety and efficacy of sonothrombolysis for acute ischaemic stroke: a multicentre, double-blind, phase 3, randomised controlled trial. Lancet Neurol. 2019;18(4):338-47.
24. Berkhemer OA, Fransen PS, Beumer D, van den Berg LA, Lingsma HF, Yoo AJ, et al.; MR CLEAN Investigators. A randomized trial of intraarterial treatment for acute ischemic stroke. N Engl J Med. 2015;372(1):11-20.
25. Goyal M, Menon BK, van Zwam WH, Dippel DW, Mitchell PJ, Demchuk AM, et al.; HERMES collaborators. Endovascular thrombectomy after large-vessel ischaemic stroke: a meta-analysis of individual patient data from five randomised trials. Lancet. 2016;387(10029):1723-31.
26. Khan A, Saqqur M, Shuaib A, Khan K, Sharma VK, Brunser A, et al.; CLOTBUST-PRO Investigators. Validation of the transcranial Doppler rescue criteria for mechanical thrombectomy. J Neuroimaging. 2024;34(4):430-7.
27. Markus HS, Droste DW, Kaps M, Larrue V, Lees KR, Siebler M, et al. Dual antiplatelet therapy with clopidogrel and aspirin in symptomatic carotid stenosis evaluated using Doppler embolic signal detection: the Clopidogrel and Aspirin for Reduction of Emboli in Symptomatic Carotid Stenosis (CARESS) trial. Circulation. 2005;111(17):2233-40.
28. Wong KS, Chen C, Fu J, Chang HM, Suwanwela NC, Huang YN, et al.; CLAIR study investigators. Clopidogrel plus aspirin versus aspirin alone for reducing embolisation in patients with acute symptomatic cerebral or carotid artery stenosis (CLAIR study): a randomised, open-label, blinded-endpoint trial. Lancet Neurol. 2010;9(5):489-97.
29. Alexandrov AV. Cerebrovascular ultrasound in stroke prevention and treatment. New York: Blackwell Publishing; 2004. pp. 81-129.
30. Lechat P, Mas JL, Lascault G, Loron P, Theard M, Klimczac M, et al. Prevalence of patent foramen ovale in patients with stroke. N Engl J Med. 1988;318(18):1148-52.
31. Anzola GP, Zavarize P, Morandi E, Rozzini L, Parrinello G. Transcranial Doppler and risk of recurrence in patients with stroke and patent foramen ovale. Eur J Neurol. 2003;10(2):129-35.
32. Belvís R, Leta RG, Martí-Fàbregas J, Cocho D, Carreras F, Pons-Lladó G, et al. Almost perfect concordance between simultaneous transcranial Doppler and transesophageal echocardiography in the quantification of right-to-left shunts. J Neuroimaging. 2006;16(2):133-8.
33. Lao AY, Sharma VK, Tsivgoulis G, Malkoff MD, Alexandrov AV, Frey JL. Effect of body positioning during transcranial Doppler detection of right-to-left shunts. Eur J Neurol. 2007;14(9):1035-9.

Recent Advances in the Management of Spontaneous Intracerebral Hemorrhage

Baikuntha Panigrahi, Ayush Agarwal

ABSTRACT

Spontaneous intracerebral hemorrhage (SICH) is the second most common cause of stroke worldwide. It is particularly common in Asians with mortality and morbidity rates higher than that of ischemic stroke. Although a devastating illness, therapeutic approaches have not paralleled advancements in ischemic stroke. The widespread nihilism has been nullified by the recent publication of quality randomized trials which have renewed optimism in managing the illness. Diagnostic advancements like the identification of iodine sign on spectral imaging have added new tools in the armamentarium of neurologists for predicting hematoma expansion. The recent boom in machine learning and artificial intelligence (AI) has provided new predictive models which are reproducible and eliminate human subjective factors. The year 2023 has reinforced therapeutic evidence by positive results of randomized controlled trials demonstrating benefits of a hyperacute care bundle approach (INTERACT3), early minimally invasive hematoma evacuation (ENRICH), and the use of Andexanet alfa in factor Xa-inhibitor anticoagulation reversal (ANNEXa-I). The current year has also added to the evidence by confirming the effects of early intensive blood pressure lowering (INTERACT4) and decompressive hemicraniectomy in large deep intracerebral hemorrhage (SWITCH). We have reviewed these and other recent developments in the management of SICH. These recent advancements usher a new positive and optimistic era for SICH care.

Keywords: Intracerebral hemorrhage, Recent advances, Hematoma expansion, Care bundles.

■ INTRODUCTION

Spontaneous intracerebral hemorrhage (SICH) is defined as rupture of cerebral blood vessels resulting in bleeding into the brain parenchyma and/or the ventricles in the absence of trauma or surgery.[1] It is the second most common cause of stroke (10–20% of all strokes) and has a pooled worldwide incidence of 29.9 per 100,000 person-years [95% confidence interval (CI) 26.5–33.3].[2] It is particularly more common in the Asian population.[2,3] The mortality rate is twice that of ischemic stroke and ranges from 40 to 50% in the 1st month.[4] The disability caused by the illness is also high with only 12–39% achieving long-term functional independence.[1] Risk factors include hypertension (HTN), age, alcohol abuse, methamphetamine or cocaine use, and presence of genetic alleles associated with cerebral amyloid angiopathy (CAA).[5] Depending on the cause, intracerebral hemorrhage (ICH) can be classified as either primary or secondary. Primary ICH accounts for about 75% of the cases and occurs due to rupture of abnormal small vessels damaged by HTN or CAA. The location of primary ICH can be lobar or nonlobar. Amyloid deposition due to CAA in the small to medium sized cortical perforators causes lobar ICH. Nonlobar ICH occurs due to lipohyalinosis of small perforators triggered by HTN. These hemorrhages are deep (often with ventricular extension) and most commonly involve the basal ganglia, thalamus, subcortical white matter, pons, and cerebellum. Secondary ICH is associated with both congenital and acquired conditions such as vascular malformations, malignancy, coagulopathies, anticoagulant and thrombolytic use, cerebral vasculitis, drug abuse, and cerebral venous thrombosis.

Even though ICH remains a major cause of morbidity and mortality, therapeutic approaches to its management over the years have not paralleled the pace of ischemic stroke. With the recent publication of quality randomized trials in the past 2 years, this nihilistic perspective has changed to an optimistic one. This article attempts to provide the reader with an updated perspective on the management of SICH in the context of recent trials.

■ DIAGNOSTIC ADVANCEMENTS IN THE CURRENT ERA

Predicting Hematoma Expansion in Intracerebral Hemorrhage

Hematoma expansion (HE) is an independent predictor of poor prognosis after an ICH and occurs in up to one-third of cases.[6] Although it has been described heterogeneously across studies, the most accepted definition across studies is an absolute increase in the volume by 6-12.5 mL and/or more than one-third of the initial volume in follow-up CT scans.[7] Numerous studies have identified specific CT, CT angiography (CTA), and MRI findings which are associated with HE and include the spot sign, leakage sign, spot-tail sign, iodine sign, island sign, satellite sign, blend sign, swirl sign, black hole sign, fluid-blood level, and MRI spot sign.[6,8-17] These signs are summarized in the **Table 1**.[18,19] Among these, the iodine sign on spectral imaging, subarachnoid extension (SAHE), and the MRI spot sign are recently described entities.

TABLE 1: Imaging signs of hematoma expansion with the description and their sensitivity, specificity, PPV, and NPV in predicting it.

Imaging	Sign	Description	Sensitivity (%)	Specificity (%)	PPV (%)	NPV (%)
CTA	Spot sign[8]	Enhanced focus in the hematoma-contrast extravasation (site of vessel rupture)	91 (62–100)	89 (72–96)	77 (50–92)	96 (81–99)
	Leakage sign[9]	Increase in CT Hounsfield value within a specific region of interest (>10%)	93.3 (75.7–98.8)	88.9 (81.5–91.2)	—	—
	Spot tail sign[10]	Presence of intrahematoma striate artery on CTA	—	—	—	—

Continued

Continued

Imaging	Sign	Description	Sensitivity (%)	Specificity (%)	PPV (%)	NPV (%)
CTA-gemstone spectral imaging (GSI)	Iodine sign[11]	Hematoma with enhancing foci on GSI + Internal focus iodine concentration of >7.82 (100 μg/mL)	91.5	79.5	82.7	89.7
NCCT	Island Sign[12]	≥3 small hematomas scattered from the main hematoma or ≥4 small hematomas with only some scattered from the main hematoma	44.7	98.2	92.7	77.7
	Satellite sign[13]	Small hematoma completely separated from the main hematoma of diameter ≤10 mm with a distance between main and small hematoma ranging from 1 to 20 mm	—	—	—	—
	Blend sign[14]	A low-density region within a region of high density within the hematoma (difference 18 HU between the two regions and low-density region not completely surrounded by high density region)	39.3	95.5	82.7	74.1
	Swirl sign[15]	Areas of hypoattenuation/isoattenuation as compared to the brain parenchyma on axial/coronal planes	—	—	—	—
	Black-hole sign[18]	Low-density area completely surrounded by high-density hematoma and a difference of at least 28 HU between them	31.9	94.1	73.3	73.2
	Fluid-blood level[6]	Horizontal interface between hypodense bloody serum and hyperdense fluid (most often seen in anticoagulant induced bleeds)	—	—	—	—
	Subarachnoid extension[19]	Predictor of lobar HE	83 (71–92)	56 (45–67)	57 (45–67)	83 (70–91)

Continued

Continued

Imaging	Sign	Description	Sensitivity (%)	Specificity (%)	PPV (%)	NPV (%)
MRI	Spot sign[17]	Spot like/serpiginous high signal >1.5 mm in one dimension located within the margins of the hematoma without any connections to any external blood vessel	90 (74–98)	47 (37–58)	94 (83–99)	35 (25–46)

(CTA: CT angiography; GSI: gemstone spectral imaging; HE: hematoma expansion; HU: hounsfield units; NCCT: noncontrast computed tomography; NPV: negative predictive value; PPV: positive predictive value)

These subjective signs have been the basis of development of scores for HE which help in risk stratification and triaging patients for a more aggressive management. The BAT, BRAIN, PREDICT-A/B, and the Brouwers 9-point score have been described which predict HE with reasonable accuracy. The salient features of each of these scores have been summarized in the **Table 2**.[20-24]

Recent Artificial Intelligence Boom and Usage in Predicting Hematoma Expansion

The advent of artificial intelligence (AI) and deep machine learning (ML) has led to better mining and integration of medical imaging information (radiomics) with clinical information (clinicomics).[25] These systems are reproducible and eliminate the human subjective factors in interpretation. Different ML models have been studied which include the k-nearest neighbors (KNN), support vector machines (SVMs), random forests, and XGBoost which have been developed using different programming languages (Python and its libraries).[26-29] Baseline clinical characteristics, ICH volume, CT and CTA imaging markers, location of the ICH, and the systolic blood pressure (SBP) have served as inputs in these algorithms with the HE as the output. In a systematic review involving 34 ML studies on HE, radiomics combined with clinical data predicted HE better than models using radiomic features or clinical features alone with a C-index of 0.79 (validation cohort) for the combined model and 0.73 (validation cohort) and 0.70 (validation cohort) in the radiomic and clinical models, respectively.[28]

DIAGRAM for Predicting Macrovascular Cause

Although in most cases, a NCCT is often enough in identifying the etiology in primary ICH (due to microvascular disease) with typical lobar and nonlobar locations as described above, certain features increase the likelihood of finding a macrovascular cause like vascular malformations. In the DIAGRAM (DIagnostic AngioGRAphy to find vascular Malformations) study, young age, lobar or posterior fossa location of ICH, and absence of small vessel disease (SVD) were associated with a significant probability of finding a macrovascular cause.[30] The usefulness is highlighted in the European Stroke Organization (ESO) 2023 expert consensus statement on use of acute care bundle in ICH which recommended the use of tools like the DIAGRAM score to identify selected patients who need further imaging like CT angiography for identifying a macrovascular cause.[31]

TABLE 2: HE prediction scores using clinical and/or radiologic data.

Score	Range	Cut-off points (risk of HE)	C-statistic/sensitivity/specificity
Brouwers score*[20]	0–9	0 (5.7%); 1–3 (12.4%); 4–9 (36.4%)	0.77 (validation cohort)
PREDICT-A$[21]	0–23	0–2 (7.1%); 15–23 (70%)	For cut off = 2; sensitivity—0.96 (0.9–0.99), specificity—0.25 (0.2–0.32)
PREDICT-B#[21]	0–28	0–5 (5.6%); 21–28 (73.3%)	For cut off = 5; sensitivity—0.97 (0.91–0.99), specificity–0.25 (0.19–0.32)
BAT[22]	0–5	0–2 (11%); 3–5 (50.8%)	2 validation cohorts—0.65 (0.61–0.68) and 0.70 (0.64–0.77)/sensitivity—50% (at score 3)/specificity—89% (at score 3)
BRAIN[23]	0–24	24 (85.8%)	C-statistic = 0.73 (INTERACT2 cohort)
Fu score@[24]	0–10	Cut-off = 3 (AUROC-0.937)	Sensitivity (at cut-off = 3)—97.8%, specificity (at cut-off = 3)—92.7%

*Brouwers score—Warfarin usage (2 points), time to NCCT (≤6 hours—2 points), CTA spot sign (present—3 points), baseline ICH volume (0–2 points).

$PREDICT-A components—GCS (0–4 points), hours to NCCT (0–5 points), Warfarin use (0–4 points), CTA spot sign number (0–8 points).

#PREDICT-B components—NIHSS (0–7 points); hours to NCCT (0–5 points), Warfarin use (0–7 points), CTA spot sign number (0–9 points).

@Fu score—Intracerebral hemorrhage baseline volume (0–1 point), time to initial NCCT ≤ 3 hours (2 points), Island sign (6 points), and black hole sign (1 point).

[AUROC: area under the receiver operating characteristic curve; BAT: B—blend sign (1 point), A—any hypodensity (2 points), T—time from onset to NCCT < 2.5 hours (2 points); BRAIN: B—baseline intracerebral hemorrhage volume (0–7 points), R—recurrent intracerebral hemorrhage (4 points), A—anticoagulation use (6 points), I—intraventricular extension (0–2 points), N—number of hours to baseline NCCT (0–5 points); HE: hematoma expansion; NCCT: noncontrast computed tomography]

■ RECENT ADVANCES IN TREATMENT OF SPONTANEOUS INTRACEREBRAL HEMORRHAGE

Treat to Target in Intracerebral Hemorrhage: Stopping the "Avalanche"

Rupture of a blood vessel inside the brain parenchyma triggers a "hemorrhagic avalanche" which causes the surrounding potentially abnormal microvessels to tear increasing the hematoma volume.[32] The initial goal of treatment should be to prevent the rupture of these microvessels and stop the avalanche. Publication of a series of randomized trials which will be discussed subsequently has provided quality Level-1 evidence for targeted interventions in the hyperacute phase (<6 hours of onset).[33] We propose a novel acronym "R-ICH" for hyperacute targets in SICH. RICH stands for *R*educe *I*njury (brain parenchyma), *C*lot burden (surgical removal), and *H*ematoma expansion.

Once the RICH targets have been achieved, postacute and long-term goals can be set. These are the two *"R"s*—recurrence prevention and rehabilitation.

RICH Goals: Care Bundles

Although care bundles are known to improve outcomes in ischemic stroke, they had not been tested in a randomized fashion in ICH.[34] Single interventions like blood pressure (BP) reduction (INTERACT2 and ATACH-2), hematoma evacuation, blood sugar, and temperature control had been tested with mixed results.[33] Combining them into a care bundle was tested in a randomized trial (INTERACT3).[35] In this international stepped wedge cluster randomized trial involving 7,036 patients of ICH presenting within 6 hours of onset, implementation of a care bundle comprising warfarin-related anticoagulation reversal (target INR < 1.5) within 1 hour, early intensive SBP control (target <140 mm Hg), care pathway for neurosurgery referral, glycemic (target in nondiabetics = 6.1–7.8 mmol/L and diabetics = 7.8–10.0 mmol/L) and temperature control (body temperature target ≤37.5°C) was associated with a lower likelihood of a poor outcome at 6 months in the care bundle group (OR 0.86; 95% CI 0.76–0.97; $p = 0.015$). The major hindrance in translating this evidence to practice is the challenges in implementation due to differential availability of resources across centers and skill mix as was seen in this study.[36] The core components of the care bundle along with the current recommended ESO and American Stroke Association/American Heart Association (ASA/AHA) guidelines are summarized in the **Table 3**.

TABLE 3: Core components of acute ICH care/care bundle with targets as per ESO/ASA/AHA guidelines.[31,37]

Intervention	Whom to treat	Door to target time	Drugs and therapeutic targets
Reversal of anticoagulation	Patients on VKA with INR ≥1.3	<30 minutes	PCC (25–50 U/kg) and vitamin K (5–10 mg)
	On apixaban or rivaroxaban and last dose taken ≤18 h		Andexanet alfa 400 mg @30 mg/min f/b 4 mg/min for 120 minutes
	On dabigatran		Idarucizumab 5 g (if available) or PCC
Intensive BP lowering	Mild-to-moderate ICHs with presenting SBP = 150–220 mm Hg	Start within 2 hours and reach target in 1 hour	Target SBP: 130–150 mm Hg; <130 mm Hg harmful
	Large ICHs with SBP > 150 mm Hg		Role of intensive SBP reduction unclear
Surgical evacuation of hematoma ± External ventricular drainage	Urgent neurosurgery consult in cases of: • GCS ≤13 • Supratentorial ICH with volume ≥ 20 mL • Posterior fossa ICH • Obstruction of 3rd and 4th ventricles	As soon as patient arrives	• MIS ± thrombolytic for GCS—5–12 and supratentorial ICH with volume ≥ 20 mL • Large IVH with hydrocephalus—EVD > medical management • GCS >3 + ICH volume < 30 mL + IVH requiring EVD→ EVD + thrombolytic • Large deep supratentorial ICHs—decompressive craniotomy • Deteriorating supratentorial ICH—craniotomy and hematoma evacuation* • Posterior fossa ICH—suboccipital decompression

Continued

Continued

Intervention	Whom to treat	Door to target time	Drugs and therapeutic targets
Glycemic control	Nondiabetics blood glucose > 7.8 mmol/L	Maintain for 7 days	Avoid hypoglycemia
	Diabetics: Blood glucose > 10 mmol/L		
Control of body temperature	Body temperature ≥37.5°C	Normothermia in < 1 hour	Temperature monitoring q4h for 7 days and any antipyretic can be used—tablet paracetamol

*Mortality benefit.
(EVD: external ventricular drain; GCS: Glasgow Coma Scale; ICH: intracerebral hemorrhage; INR: international normalized ratio; IVH: intraventricular hemorrhage; MIS: minimally invasive surgery; PCC: prothrombin complex concentrate; SBP: systolic blood pressure; VKA: vitamin K antagonists)

Time is Brain in ICH Too!

In May 2024, the INTERACT4 was published which randomly assigned 2,404 acute stroke patients (both ischemic and hemorrhagic) with a motor deficit and elevated SBP (≥150 mm Hg), within 2 hours after the onset of symptoms assessed in the ambulance, to receive immediate treatment to lower the SBP (target range = 130–140 mm Hg; intervention group) or usual BP control.[38] Although there was no difference in functional outcomes between the two groups, the intervention group was associated with decreased odds of poor functional outcome among patients with ICH (common odds ratio 0.75; 95% CI 0.60–0.92). These novel findings underscore the benefits of rapid BP control (<2 hours) in ICH patients and provide evidence for reconfiguring current systems of care for a time intensive urgency toward BP reduction.[33]

ANTICOAGULATION REVERSAL: RECENT ADVANCES

- *The increasing use of direct oral anticoagulants (DOACs) and challenges in ICH treatment*: In a recent Italian population-based stroke registry study, although the incidence of oral anticoagulation related ICH remained stable over a decade, the incidence of DOAC-related ICH overtook that related to vitamin K antagonists (VKA) in 2020 (incidence rate ratio 4.71; 95% CI 1.22–33.54; $p=0.022$).[39] Similar Indian studies are needed to substantiate this claim. The ease-of-use of DOACs makes them preferable to VKAs. However, unlike rapid reversal agents and ability to monitor for overdose for VKAs (INCH trial), DOAC antidotes have not been previously tested in a randomized fashion.[40] In a prospective cohort study (RE-VERSE AD) evaluating a specific agent to reverse the anticoagulant effects of dabigatran involving 90 patients, idarucizumab normalized test results (dilute thrombin time or ecarin clotting time) in 88–98% of the patients, an effect that was evident within minutes at a dose of 5 g intravenously.[41] Whether these results translate to improved functional outcomes in dabigatran-induced ICH patients remains unexplored. Idarucizumab has recently been introduced in India, but the high costs preclude its widespread use.[42]

- *Tranexamic acid and novel oral anticoagulant induced ICH (NOAC-ICH)*: The efficacy of the antifibrinolytic drug tranexamic acid was tested in a randomized trial (TICH-NOAC) involving 63 patients (32 in IV tranexamic acid arm and 31 in the placebo arm) of NOAC-ICH within 48 hours of NOAC intake and 12 hours of onset of symptoms. The primary outcome of HE was not significantly different between the two arms (aOR 0.63; 95% CI 0.22–1.82; $p = 0.40$).[43] Although the trial did not reach its intended sample size of 109 patients which precludes any firm conclusions, it was the first randomized trial for hemostatic treatments in NOAC-ICH.
- *ANNEXing andexanet alfa into the armamentarium*: Factor Xa inhibitors (FXaI) present a different challenge and have been treated with prothrombin complex concentrates mainly based on observational data.[44] However, the introduction of andexanet alfa, a recombinant modified factor Xa antidote which acts as a decoy and sequesters factor Xa inhibitors, resulted in a targeted therapy for FXaI-ICH. In an individual patient level meta-analysis of the ANNEXa-4 and the TICH-NOAC studies, treatment with andexanet alfa was independently associated with decreased odds of HE (aOR 0.33; 95% CI 0.13–0.80; $p = 0.015$) compared to a nonspecific treatment strategy.[45]

The ANNEXa-I further strengthened evidence in favor of andexanet alfa. In this randomized trial involving 452 patients for efficacy analysis, the primary endpoint of hemostatic efficacy occurred in 67% of patients receiving andexanet and in 53.1% patients receiving usual care (adjusted difference = 13.4 percentage points; 95% CI 4.6–22.2; $p = 0.003$).[46] There was, however, an associated increase in thrombotic events including ischemic stroke (thrombotic events in 10.3% of patients in the andexanet arm as compared to 5.6% usual care arm; difference = 4.6 percentage points; 95% CI 0.1–9.2; $p = 0.048$); ischemic stroke occurred in 6.5% versus 1.5% patients, respectively. The trial was not powered to show a difference in mortality or functional outcomes, the question which still remains unanswered.

ADVANCES IN SURGICAL MANAGEMENT OF INTRACEREBRAL HEMORRHAGE

The choice of patients for surgical treatment, the most appropriate technique, and the optimal timing of intervention have been a matter of debate for years.[47] This is primarily due to randomized trials failing to demonstrate any benefit of hematoma evacuation on death and functional outcome compared to conservative care.

In supratentorial ICH patients with a hematoma volume >10 mL and significant neurological deficit, the benefits of craniotomy compared to conservative management remain uncertain.[37] Both the STICH I and STICH II failed to demonstrate any improvement in functional outcomes with craniotomy.[48,49] Limited data, however, suggests that craniotomy for hematoma evacuation may be considered in deteriorating patients as a lifesaving measure primarily due to the STICH II identifying a trend toward decreased mortality with surgery, despite a crossover rate of 21% from conservative arm to surgery of which 74% were attributable to deterioration.[49]

In the recent years, there has been interest in minimally invasive surgery (MIS) for hematoma evacuation in supratentorial ICHs using endoscopic or stereotactic aspiration mainly due to its propensity to reduce hematoma volume, perihematomal edema, and less destruction of brain tissue as compared to conventional craniotomy.[37] However, this enthusiasm had not translated into trial results until the ENRICH results.[50] In the MISTIE-III (Third Minimally Invasive Surgery with Thrombolysis in Intracerebral Hemorrhage Evacuation) trial involving 499 patients (255 in the MISTIE arm and 251 in the usual medical care arm-modified intention to treat), no overall benefit was seen in the primary outcome of functional recovery in the MIS group with local application of alteplase for hematoma aspiration within 6-72 hours after onset (adjusted risk difference = 4%; 95% CI 4-12; $p = 0.33$).[51]

The ENRICH trial looked at whether early MIS resulted in better functional outcomes compared to medical management.[50] In this study involving 300 patients (150 in surgical arm and 150 in medical arm) of lobar (69.3%) or anterior basal ganglia (30.7%) ICH with a hematoma volume of 30-80 mL within 24 hours after the time last known to be well, MIS resulted in better functional outcomes at 180 days which was primarily due to intervention for lobar ICHs. Although this trial supported MIS surgery for lobar supratentorial ICHs, it left several questions unanswered over the optimal technique and patient selection for early surgery. Further ongoing trials like the NESICH (NCT05539859), MIND (NCT03342664), EVACUATE (NCT04434807), DIST (NCT05460793), and EMINENT-ICH (NCT05681988) will provide better answers to the optimal timing, technique, and the right patient for MIS.[33,52]

TIME TO SWITCH TO DECOMPRESSIVE CRANIECTOMY FOR LARGE DEEP SUPRATENTORIAL INTRA-CEREBRAL HEMORRHAGES?

Until 2024, it was unknown if decompressive craniectomy led to improved clinical outcomes in severe deep ICHs. The SWITCH was a multicenter, open label assessor blinded randomized trial involving 197 patients (96 in decompressive craniectomy plus usual care and 101 in usual care) which suggested that decompressive craniectomy plus usual care might be superior to usual care alone in patients with large deep supratentorial ICHs (adjusted risk difference −13%; 95% CI −26 to 0).[53] Further large trials are needed to substantiate these results.

POST-INTRACEREBRAL HEMORRHAGES CARE

Enhancing post ICH recovery is an area of active research. Most rehabilitative strategies have focused on gross motor recovery neglecting the sensory and the cognitive aspects of the deficit. Recently, numerous lower limb exoskeletons have been developed for assisting or augmenting with walking. Some of them are stationary and are used mainly for gait retraining after trauma. Others are mobile and support the entire body weight or provide an assistive force while walking. In a randomized trial of exoskeleton-based physical therapy (ExStRA) involving 36 patients with a median of 39 days post stroke (both ischemic and hemorrhagic stroke included), no significant improvement in walking independence (functional ambulation category) was found as compared to standard care.[54] The development of Robotics has led to development of Robotic mobile exoskeletons for gait training of stroke survivors.

The timing of rehabilitation is also a matter of debate with studies suggesting that very early and intensive rehabilitation can impair functional recovery.[55] The AHA/ASA 2022 guideline recommends that rehabilitation should be started 24–48 hours after stroke onset. In addition, it recommended against intense and frequent mobilization within 24 hours. In remote areas, there has been increasing enthusiasm in the field of telerehabilitation with randomized trials demonstrating low-to-

CHAPTER 2: Recent Advances in the Management of Spontaneous Intracerebral Hemorrhage

moderate evidence that they are noninferior to in-person care.[56,57]

Depression is also common following ICH and may occur in up to 20% of patients. The benefits of treatment must be balanced by the increased risk of secondary events with selective serotonin reuptake inhibitors. Three recent randomized trials (FOCUS, AFFINITY, and EFFECTS) tried to harness the pleiotropic effects of fluoxetine enrolling both ischemic

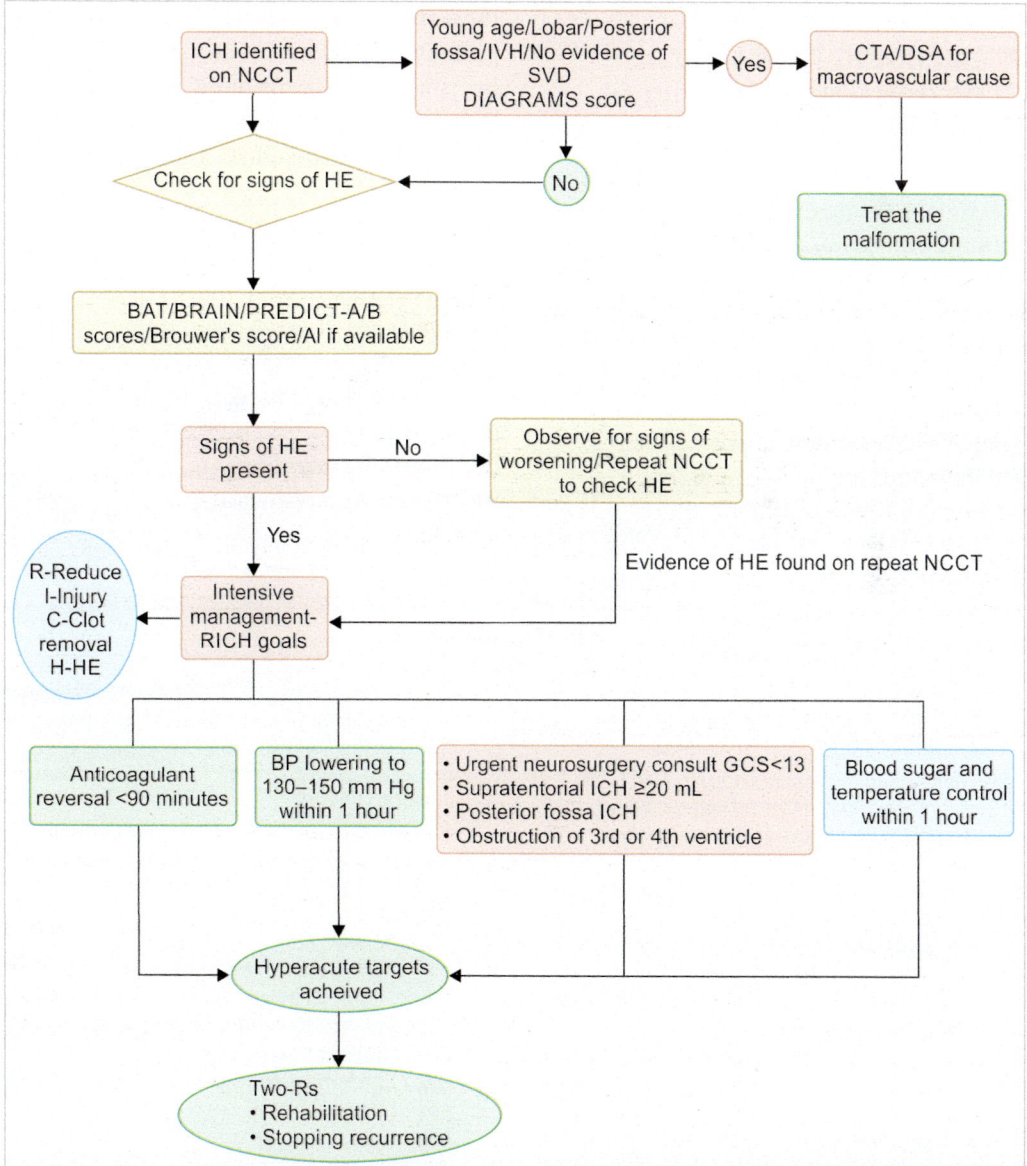

FLOWCHART 1: Management algorithm for spontaneous ICH in the current era with emphasis on time bound targets.

(ICH: intracerebral hemorrhage; NCCT: noncontrast computed tomography scan; SVD: small vessel disease; HE: hematoma expansion)

stroke and ICH patients and found that, although the risk of poststroke depression was reduced, the risk of bone fractures and hyponatremia was increased, and no significant improvements in functional outcomes were seen.[58]

EMERGING THERAPEUTIC OPTIONS: NANOPARTICLES

Recently, numerous active pharmaceutical ingredients have been used in ICH mainly in preclinical studies which include desferoxamine, curcumin, and resveratrol.[59] These drugs target ferroptosis and the oxidative stress. The major issue precluding their use has been their toxicity and poor bioavailability. Nanotechnology has allowed us a novel method of drug loading enhancing target bioavailability. Nanomaterials such as polymer, micelles, nanoemulsions, liposomes, and exosomes have been recently tried in ICH and have shown promise. Further developments in nanotechnology might make randomized studies feasible in the coming decade.

CONCLUSION

As seen in this review, there has been an increase in the intensity in managing ICH patients which has been primarily driven by the above-mentioned positive trials. Enlightened by the RICH and double-R approach, we propose a new algorithm for managing ICH in the current era incorporating evidence gained from these studies **(Flowchart 1)**. As we eagerly wait for the results of ongoing trials to further change the ICH landscape, time has come to shift gears to a more intensive "Time is brain" approach. Emerging advancements in diagnostics using AI and therapeutics using nanoparticles are likely to further reduce morbidity and mortality in the coming decade.

REFERENCES

1. An SJ, Kim TJ, Yoon BW. Epidemiology, Risk Factors, and Clinical Features of Intracerebral Hemorrhage: An Update. J Stroke. 2017;19(1):3-10.
2. Wang S, Zou XL, Wu LX, Zhou HF, Xiao L, Yao T, et al. Epidemiology of intracerebral hemorrhage: A systematic review and meta-analysis. Front Neurol. 2022;13:915813.
3. Van Asch CJ, Luitse MJ, Rinkel GJ, Van Der Tweel I, Algra A, Klijn CJ. Incidence, case fatality, and functional outcome of intracerebral haemorrhage over time, according to age, sex, and ethnic origin: a systematic review and meta-analysis. Lancet Neurol. 2010;9(2):167-76.
4. Woo D, Comeau ME, Venema SU, Anderson CD, Flaherty M, Testai F, et al. Risk Factors Associated With Mortality and Neurologic Disability After Intracerebral Hemorrhage in a Racially and Ethnically Diverse Cohort. JAMA Netw Open. 2022;5(3):e221103.
5. Dastur CK, Yu W. Current management of spontaneous intracerebral haemorrhage. Stroke Vasc Neurol. 2017;2(1):21-9.
6. Huang YW, Huang HL, Li ZP, Yin XS. Research advances in imaging markers for predicting hematoma expansion in intracerebral hemorrhage: a narrative review. Front Neurol. 2023;14:1176390.
7. Haupenthal D, Schwab S, Kuramatsu JB. Hematoma expansion in intracerebral hemorrhage – the right target? Neurol Res Pract. 2023;5(1):36.
8. Wada R, Aviv RI, Fox AJ, Sahlas DJ, Gladstone DJ, Tomlinson G, et al. CT Angiography "Spot Sign" Predicts Hematoma Expansion in Acute Intracerebral Hemorrhage. Stroke. 2007;38(4):1257-62.
9. Orito K, Hirohata M, Nakamura Y, Takeshige N, Aoki T, Hattori G, et al. Leakage Sign for Primary Intracerebral Hemorrhage: A Novel Predictor of Hematoma Growth. Stroke. 2016;47(4):958-63.
10. Sorimachi T, Osada T, Baba T, Inoue G, Atsumi H, Ishizaka H, et al. The Striate Artery, Hematoma, and Spot Sign on Coronal Images of Computed Tomography Angiography in

Putaminal Intracerebral Hemorrhage. Stroke. 2013;44(7):1830-2.
11. Fu F, Sun S, Liu L, Gu H, Su Y, Li Y. Iodine Sign as a Novel Predictor of Hematoma Expansion and Poor Outcomes in Primary Intracerebral Hemorrhage Patients. Stroke. 2018;49(9):2074-80.
12. Li Q, Liu QJ, Yang WS, Wang XC, Zhao LB, Xiong X, et al. Island Sign: An Imaging Predictor for Early Hematoma Expansion and Poor Outcome in Patients with Intracerebral Hemorrhage. Stroke. 2017;48(11):3019-25.
13. Shimoda Y, Ohtomo S, Arai H, Okada K, Tominaga T. Satellite Sign: A Poor Outcome Predictor in Intracerebral Hemorrhage. Cerebrovasc Dis. 2017;44(3-4):105-12.
14. Li Q, Zhang G, Huang YJ, Dong MX, Lv FJ, Wei X, et al. Blend Sign on Computed Tomography: Novel and Reliable Predictor for Early Hematoma Growth in Patients With Intracerebral Hemorrhage. Stroke. 2015;46(8):2119-23.
15. Al-Nakshabandi NA. The Swirl Sign. Radiology. 2001;218(2):433.
16. Suzuki R, Yamasaki T, Koizumi S, Nozaki T, Hiramatsu H, Sameshima T, et al. Fluid-Blood Level and Hematoma Expansion in a Cerebral Amyloid Angiopathy-Associated Intracerebral Hematoma. Am J Case Rep. 2019;20:844-50.
17. Valyraki N, Goujon A, Mateos M, Lecoeuvre A, Lecler A, Raynouard I, et al. MRI spot sign in acute intracerebral hemorrhage: an independent biomarker of hematoma expansion and poor functional outcome. J Neurol. 2023;270(3):1531-42.
18. Li Q, Zhang G, Xiong X, Wang XC, Yang WS, Li KW, et al. Black Hole Sign: Novel Imaging Marker That Predicts Hematoma Growth in Patients with Intracerebral Hemorrhage. Stroke. 2016;47(7):1777-81.
19. Morotti A, Poli L, Leuci E, Mazzacane F, Costa P, De Giuli V, et al. Subarachnoid Extension Predicts Lobar Intracerebral Hemorrhage Expansion. Stroke. 2020;51(5):1470-6.
20. Brouwers HB, Chang Y, Falcone GJ, Cai X, Ayres AM, Battey TW, et al. Predicting Hematoma Expansion after Primary Intracerebral Hemorrhage. JAMA Neurol. 2014;71(2):158-64.
21. Huynh TJ, Aviv RI, Dowlatshahi D, Gladstone DJ, Laupacis A, Kiss A, et al. Validation of the 9-Point and 24-Point Hematoma Expansion Prediction Scores and Derivation of the PREDICT A/B Scores. Stroke. 2015;46(11):3105-10.
22. Morotti A, Dowlatshahi D, Boulouis G, Al-Ajlan F, Demchuk AM, Aviv RI, et al. Predicting Intracerebral Hemorrhage Expansion With Noncontrast Computed Tomography: The BAT Score. Stroke. 2018;49(5):1163-9.
23. Wang X, Arima H, Al-Shahi Salman R, Woodward M, Heeley E, Stapf C, et al. Clinical Prediction Algorithm (BRAIN) to Determine Risk of Hematoma Growth in Acute Intracerebral Hemorrhage. Stroke. 2015;46(2):376-81.
24. Fu J, Hu S, Yang M, Li Z, Song X, Wang Z, et al. A Novel 10-Point Score System to Predict Early Hematoma Growth in Patients with Spontaneous Intracerebral Hemorrhage. Front Neurol. 2020;10:1417.
25. Van Timmeren JE, Cester D, Tanadini-Lang S, Alkadhi H, Baessler B. Radiomics in medical imaging—"how-to" guide and critical reflection. Insights Imaging. 2020;11(1):91.
26. Tang ZR, Chen Y, Hu R, Wang H. Predicting hematoma expansion in intracerebral hemorrhage from brain CT scans via K-nearest neighbors matting and deep residual network. Biomed Signal Process Control. 2022;76:103656.
27. Liu J, Xu H, Chen Q, Zhang T, Sheng W, Huang Q, et al. Prediction of hematoma expansion in spontaneous intracerebral hemorrhage using support vector machine. EBioMedicine. 2019;43:454-9.
28. Liu Y, Zhao F, Niu E, Chen L. Machine learning for predicting hematoma expansion in spontaneous intracerebral hemorrhage: a systematic review and meta-analysis. Neuroradiology. 2024;66(9):1603-16.
29. Tanioka S, Yago T, Tanaka K, Ishida F, Kishimoto T, Tsuda K, et al. Machine learning prediction of hematoma expansion in acute intracerebral hemorrhage. Sci Rep. 2022;12(1):12452.
30. Hilkens NA, Van Asch CJJ, Werring DJ, Wilson D, Rinkel GJE, Algra A, et al. Predicting the presence of macrovascular causes in non-traumatic intracerebral haemorrhage: the DIAGRAM prediction score. J Neurol Neurosurg Psychiatry. 2018;89(7):674-9.
31. Parry-Jones AR, Järhult SJ, Kreitzer N, Morotti A, Toni D, Seiffge D, et al. Acute care bundles should be used for patients with intracerebral haemorrhage: An expert consensus statement. Eur Stroke J. 2024;9(2):295-302.
32. Veltkamp R, Purrucker J. Management of Spontaneous Intracerebral Hemorrhage. Curr Neurol Neurosci Rep. 2017;17(10):80.
33. Seiffge DJ, Anderson CS. Treatment for intracerebral hemorrhage: Dawn of a new era. Int J Stroke. 2024;19(5):482-9.

34. Middleton S, McElduff P, Ward J, Grimshaw JM, Dale S, D'Este C, et al. Implementation of evidence-based treatment protocols to manage fever, hyperglycaemia, and swallowing dysfunction in acute stroke (QASC): a cluster randomised controlled trial. Lancet. 2011;378(9804):1699-706.
35. Ma L, Hu X, Song L, Chen X, Ouyang M, Billot L, et al. The third Intensive Care Bundle with Blood Pressure Reduction in Acute Cerebral Haemorrhage Trial (INTERACT3): an international, stepped wedge cluster randomised controlled trial. Lancet. 2023;402(10395):27-40.
36. Ouyang M, Anderson CS, Song L, Jan S, Sun L, Cheng G, et al. Implementing a Goal-Directed Care Bundle after Acute Intracerebral Haemorrhage: Process Evaluation for the Third INTEnsive Care Bundle with Blood Pressure Reduction in Acute Cerebral Haemorrhage Trial Study in China. Cerebrovasc Dis. 2022;51(3):373-83.
37. Greenberg SM, Ziai WC, Cordonnier C, Dowlatshahi D, Francis B, Goldstein JN, et al. 2022 Guideline for the Management of Patients with Spontaneous Intracerebral Hemorrhage: A Guideline From the American Heart Association/American Stroke Association. Stroke. 2022;53(7):e282-e361.
38. Li G, Lin Y, Yang J, Anderson CS, Chen C, Liu F, et al. Intensive Ambulance-Delivered Blood-Pressure Reduction in Hyperacute Stroke. N Engl J Med. 2024;390(20):1862-72.
39. Gabriele F, Foschi M, Conversi F, Ciuffini D, De Santis F, Orlandi B, et al. Epidemiology and outcomes of intracerebral hemorrhage associated with oral anticoagulation over 10 years in a population-based stroke registry. Int J Stroke. 2024;19(5):515-25.
40. Steiner T, Poli S, Griebe M, Hüsing J, Hajda J, Freiberger A, et al. Fresh frozen plasma versus prothrombin complex concentrate in patients with intracranial haemorrhage related to vitamin K antagonists (INCH): a randomised trial. Lancet Neurol. 2016;15(6):566-73.
41. Pollack CV, Reilly PA, Eikelboom J, Glund S, Verhamme P, Bernstein RA, et al. Idarucizumab for Dabigatran Reversal. N Engl J Med. 2015;373(6):511-20.
42. Mashru M, Shah MS, Shah AB, Kalra S, Bhapkar S. Successful use of idarucizumab for the management of intracranial hemorrhage in an elderly woman receiving dabigatran for stroke prevention in atrial fibrillation: A case report. IHJ Cardiovasc Case Rep. 2018;2(3):166-8.
43. Polymeris AA, Karwacki GM, Siepen BM, Schaedelin S, Tsakiris DA, Stippich C, et al. Tranexamic Acid for Intracerebral Hemorrhage in Patients on Non-Vitamin K Antagonist Oral Anticoagulants (TICH-NOAC): A Multicenter, Randomized, Placebo-Controlled, Phase 2 Trial. Stroke. 2023;54(9):2223-34.
44. Panos NG, Cook AM, John S, Jones GM; Neurocritical Care Society (NCS) Pharmacy Study Group. Factor Xa Inhibitor-Related Intracranial Hemorrhage: Results From a Multicenter, Observational Cohort Receiving Prothrombin Complex Concentrates. Circulation. 2020;141(21):1681-9.
45. Siepen BM, Polymeris A, Shoamanesh A, Connolly S, Steiner T, Poli S, et al. Andexanet alfa versus non-specific treatments for intracerebral hemorrhage in patients taking factor Xa inhibitors—Individual patient data analysis of ANNEXA-4 and TICH-NOAC. Int J Stroke. 2024;19(5):506-14.
46. Connolly SJ, Sharma M, Cohen AT, Demchuk AM, Członkowska A, Lindgren AG, et al. Andexanet for Factor Xa Inhibitor–Associated Acute Intracerebral Hemorrhage. N Engl J Med. 2024;390(19):1745-55.
47. Dammers R, Beck J, Volovici V, Anderson CS, Klijn CJM. Advancing the Surgical Treatment of Intracerebral Hemorrhage: Study Design and Research Directions. World Neurosurg. 2022;161:367-75.
48. Mendelow A, Gregson B, Fernandes H, Murray GD, Teasdale GM, Hope DT, et al. Early surgery versus initial conservative treatment in patients with spontaneous supratentorial intracerebral haematomas in the International Surgical Trial in Intracerebral Haemorrhage (STICH): a randomised trial. Lancet. 2005;365(9457):387-97.
49. Mendelow AD, Gregson BA, Rowan EN, Murray GD, Gholkar A, Mitchell PM. Early surgery versus initial conservative treatment in patients with spontaneous supratentorial lobar intracerebral haematomas (STICH II): a randomised trial. Lancet. 2013;382(9890):397-408.
50. Pradilla G, Ratcliff JJ, Hall AJ, Saville BR, Allen JW, Paulon G, et al. Trial of Early Minimally Invasive Removal of Intracerebral Hemorrhage. N Engl J Med. 2024;390(14):1277-89.
51. Hanley DF, Thompson RE, Rosenblum M, Yenokyan G, Lane K, McBee N, et al. Efficacy and safety of minimally invasive surgery with thrombolysis in intracerebral haemorrhage evacuation (MISTIE III): a randomised, controlled, open-label, blinded endpoint phase 3 trial. Lancet. 2019;393(10175):1021-32.
52. Wang L, Zhou T, Wang P, Zhang S, Yin Y, Chen L, et al. Efficacy and safety of NeuroEndoscopic Surgery for IntraCerebral Hemorrhage: A randomized, controlled, open-label, blinded endpoint trial (NESICH). Int J Stroke. 2024;19(5):587-92.

53. Beck J, Fung C, Strbian D, Bütikofer L, J Z'Graggen W, Lang MF, et al. Decompressive craniectomy plus best medical treatment versus best medical treatment alone for spontaneous severe deep supratentorial intracerebral haemorrhage: a randomised controlled clinical trial. Lancet. 2024;403(10442):2395-404.
54. Louie DR, Mortenson WB, Durocher M, Schneeberg A, Teasell R, Yao J, et al. Efficacy of an exoskeleton-based physical therapy program for non-ambulatory patients during subacute stroke rehabilitation: a randomized controlled trial. J Neuroeng Rehabil. 2021;18(1):149.
55. Langhorne P, Wu O, Rodgers H, Ashburn A, Bernhardt J. A Very Early Rehabilitation Trial after stroke (AVERT): a Phase III, multicentre, randomised controlled trial. Health Technol Assess. 2017;21(54):1-120.
56. Laver KE, Adey-Wakeling Z, Crotty M, Lannin NA, George S, Sherrington C. Telerehabilitation services for stroke. Cochrane Database Syst Rev. 2020;1(1):CD010255.
57. Duncan PW, Bernhardt J. Telerehabilitation: Has Its Time Come? Stroke. 2021;52(8):2694-6.
58. Zille M, Farr TD, Keep RF, Römer C, Xi G, Boltze J. Novel targets, treatments, and advanced models for intracerebral haemorrhage. eBioMedicine. 2022;76:103880.
59. Wang J, Wang T, Fang M, Wang Z, Xu W, Teng B, et al. Advances of nanotechnology for intracerebral hemorrhage therapy. Front Bioeng Biotechnol. 2023;11:1265153.

CHAPTER 3

Advances in Intravenous Thrombolysis

Rajesh Kumar Singh, Kameshwar Prasad

ABSTRACT

Stroke is second major cause of disability and fourth most common cause of mortality in India. In 1995, the National Institute of Neurological Disorders and Stroke (NINDS) recombinant tissue plasminogen activator (rtPA) stroke trial first established the benefit of intravenous thrombolysis (IVT) with rtPA for acute ischemic stroke of duration up to 3 hours. Subsequently, the time window for thrombolysis with alteplase has been extended to 4.5 hours after European Cooperative Acute Stroke Study (ECASS)-III randomized controlled trial (RCT) and in certain circumstances even up to 9 hours based on advanced imaging. Tenecteplase (TNK) was bioengineered from rtPA and has higher fibrin specificity (14 times), longer half-life (approximately 18 minutes) and has 80 times enhanced resistance to plasminogen activator inhibitor-1 (PAI-1) leading to lesser adverse effects than alteplase. TNK has been used up to 24 hours with the help of advanced imaging with favorable outcome; thus, expanding the window period of IVT. At present, there is enough evidence from randomized trials to prove noninferiority of TNK over alteplase for acute ischemic stroke in terms of efficacy and safety. However, some observational studies suggest superiority of TNK over alteplase, yet to be confirmed in RCT. For patients with large vessel occlusion (LVO) acute ischemic stroke, direct endovascular therapy is likely noninferior to bridging therapy. However, most of bridging trials have use alteplase as the thrombolytic agent. If a superior thrombolytic agent becomes established in terms of safety and efficacy, then bridging trials may yield different results. Newer intravenous thrombolytic agents such as reteplase have shown favorable results in terms of safety and efficacy.

Keywords: Alteplase, Tenecteplase, Reteplase, Intravenous thrombolysis, Endovascular therapy, Bridging therapy.

■ INTRODUCTION

Stroke is fifth leading cause of disability and fourth leading cause of mortality in India. The burden of stroke is increasing in India and incidence ranges from 105 to 152/100,000 people per year.[1] In 1995, the National Institute of Neurological Disorders and Stroke (NINDS) recombinant tissue plasminogen activator (rtPA) Stroke trial first established the benefit of intravenous thrombolysis (IVT) with rtPA for acute ischemic stroke of duration up to 3 hours.[2] Since then, there has been many modifications in IVT with respect to drugs, dosage and time window. Many of previous contraindications for IVT have also been modified with extension of therapeutic indications.

ALTEPLASE

Time Window up to 3 Hours

The NINDS trial introduced alteplase with time window of 3 hours in acute ischemic stroke showing favorable outcome with 18% relative risk reduction (control group risk of 74% to alteplase group risk of 61%) or 13% absolute risk reduction in significant disability. Though there was significant increase in symptomatic intracranial hemorrhage (sICH) (6.4% vs. 0.6%, $p < 0.001$) but without any significant effect on mortality.[2] The benefit of IV rtPA within 3 hours is well established from multiple trials for adult patients with disabling stroke symptoms regardless of age and stroke severity. European Cooperative Acute Stroke Study (ECASS)-I[3] and ECASS-II[4] included patients of acute ischemic stroke up to 6 hours of symptom onset. Though ECASS-I and ECASS-II results failed to prove efficacy of alteplase over control but meta-analysis[5] of individual patient data supported the efficacy and safety of rtPA. Prasad et al.[6] reconducted meta-analysis with modified Rankin scale (mRS) 2 to 6 as the effect measure using the data reported in Cochrane review[7] and the forest plot is given in **Figure 1**. Examination of the summary point estimate in **Figure 1** shows that if RR is used, the relative risk reduction is 12% (**Fig. 1**).

Time Window from 3 to 4.5 Hours

ATLANTIS study randomized 613 acute ischemic strokes between 3 and 5 hours of symptom onset but it found no significant benefit of rtPA on the 90-day efficacy endpoints.[8] In 2008, ECASS-III randomized controlled trial (RCT) reported the benefit of IVT in poststroke time window of 3.0–4.5 hours. Treatment with rtPA led to more favorable outcome with more sICH (2.4% vs. 0.8%, $p = 0.008$) but with similar mortality as compared to placebo.[9] However, ECASS-III excluded octogenarians, patients taking warfarin regardless of international normalized ratio (INR) value, patients with very severe stroke (NIHSS score > 25) and diabetes. However, there was baseline imbalance in some prognostic factors, which on reanalysis explained the observed differences and adjusting for these differences revealed no difference between the alteplase and control groups.[10] However, individual patient data meta-analysis supported efficacy of alteplase up to 4.5 hours since onset.[11]

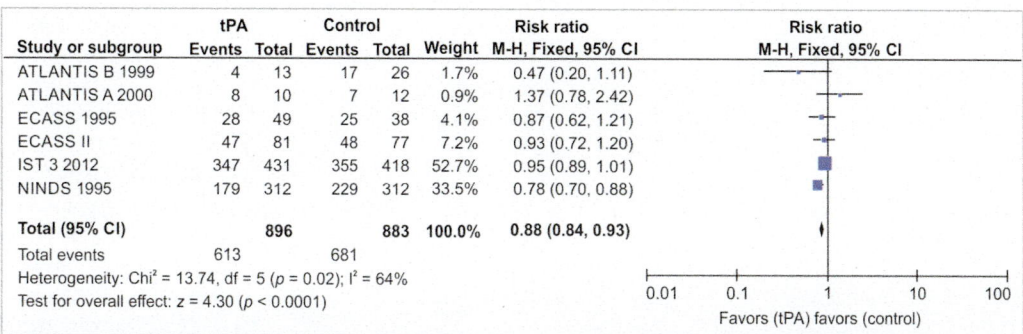

FIG. 1: Outcome: Significant disability (mRS 2–6), comparison: rtPA versus control, (within 3 hours to onset), effect measure: relative risk.

(mRS: modified Rankin scale; rtPA: recombinant tissue plasminogen activator)

Time Window from 4.5 to 9 Hours

Some trials have looked for extension of time window for IVT and suggested that it may be extended in patients who have salvageable tissue demonstrated by perfusion-diffusion mismatch. Extending the time for Thrombolysis in Emergency Neurological Deficits (EXTEND) trial randomized patients to receive intravenous alteplase or placebo between 4.5 and 9 hours after onset of stroke or on awakening with stroke (if within 9 hours from midpoint of sleep).[12] The primary outcome at 3 months (mRS 0 or 1) occurred in 40 patients (35.4%) in alteplase group and in 33 patients (29.5%) in placebo group [adjusted risk ratio (RR) 1.44; 95% confidence interval (CI) 1.01–2.06; $p = 0.04$] with development of sICH in seven patients (6.2%) in the alteplase group. Two more trials, the Echoplanar Imaging Thrombolytic Evaluation Trial (EPITHET) and ECASS-IV: EXTEND looked for extending the therapeutic window of alteplase.[13,14] EPITHET showed that alteplase group had lower infarct growth though it was statistically not significant. ECASS-IV trial also showed better outcome in alteplase group although the results were statistically non-significant. A meta-analysis of individual patient data from above three trials including 429 patients in alteplase and 414 in placebo group showed no statistically significant difference in functional outcome [odds ratio (OR) 1.38; CI 1.05–1.80, $p = 0.19$] at 3 months.[15]

■ TENECTEPLASE

Tenecteplase (TNK) was bioengineered from rtPA in which three mutations in amino acid sequences resulted in higher fibrin specificity (14 times) and longer half-life (approximately 18 minutes) leading to single bolus IV administration.[16] It has 80 times enhanced resistance to plasminogen activator inhibitor-1 (PAI-1) leading to lesser adverse effects than alteplase. It was approved for acute myocardial infarction in 2000.[17] In 2005, phase 2 study was conducted showing safety of TNK at doses of 0.1–0.4 mg/kg for ischemic stroke.[18] Many RCT have been reported subsequently comparing efficacy and safety of TNK with alteplase **(Table 1)**.[19-26]

TABLE 1: RCTs comparing efficacy and safety of tenecteplase with alteplase or placebo/standard treatment.

Trial	Design	Time window (hour)	Comparison	Patient number	Results
Parsons et al.[19] (Australian TNK 2012)	Multicenter PROBE	<6	• TNK 0.1 and 0.25 mg/kg • Alteplase 0.9 mg/kg	• TNK 50 • Alteplase 25	TNK (0.1 or 0.25 mg/kg) was associated with better reperfusion (79.3% vs. 55.4%, $p = 0.004$) and clinical improvement in NIHSS at 24 hours (8 vs. 3, $p < 0.001$) than rtPA
Huang et al.[20] (ATTEST 2015)	Multicenter PROBE	<4.5	• TNK 0.25 mg/kg • Alteplase 0.9 mg/kg	• TNK 52 • Alteplase 52	No significant differences for % of penumbral salvaged [68% (SD 28) for the TNK group vs. 68%[23] for the alteplase group; mean difference 1.3% (95% CI–9.6 to 12.1); $p = 0.81$]

Continued

Continued

Trial	Design	Time window (hour)	Comparison	Patient number	Results
Logallo et al.[21] (NOR-TEST 2017)	Multicenter PROBE superiority trial	<4.5	• TNK 0.4 mg/kg • Alteplase 0.9 mg/kg	• TNK 549 • Alteplase 551	Excellent functional outcome (mRS 0–1) at 3 months was achieved by 354 (64%) patients in the TNK group and 345 (63%) patients in the alteplase group (odds ratio 1.08; 95% CI 0.84–1.38; $p = 0.52$)
Campbell et al.[22] (EXTEND-1A TNK 2018)	Multicenter PROBE non-inferiority trial	<4.5	• TNK 0.25 mg/kg • Alteplase 0.9 mg/kg	$n = 101$	TNK before thrombectomy was associated with a higher incidence of reperfusion (22% vs. 10%, $p = 0.03$) and better functional outcome (mean mRS, 2 vs. 3, $p = 0.04$) than rtPA
Campbell et al.[23] (EXTEND-1A TNK Part 2, 2020)	Multicenter PROBE	<4.5	• TNK 0.40 mg/kg • TNK 0.25 mg/kg		EXTEND-IA TNK part 2 trial further confirmed that a dose of 0.40 mg/kg, compared with 0.25 mg/kg, of TNK did not significantly improve cerebral reperfusion prior to EVT
Menon et al.[24] (AcT 2022)	Multicenter PROBE	<4.5	• TNK 0.25 mg/kg • Alteplase 0.9 mg/kg	• TNK 816 • Alteplase 784	296 (36.9%) of 802 patients in the tenecteplase group and 266 (34.8%) of 765 in the alteplase group had an mRS score of 0–1 at 90–120 days [unadjusted risk difference 2.1% (95% CI –2.6 to 6.9), meeting the prespecified noninferiority threshold]
Albers GW et al.[25] (TIMELESS 2024)	Multicenter, double-blind, randomized, placebo-controlled trial	4.5–24	• TNK 0.25 mg/kg • Placebo	• TNK 228 • Placebo 230	The adjusted common odds ratio for the distribution of scores on the mRS at 90 days for TNK as compared with placebo was 1.13 (95% CI; 0.82–1.57; $p = 0.45$). It did not result in better clinical outcomes than those with placebo

Continued

Continued

Trial	Design	Time window (hour)	Comparison	Patient number	Results
Xiong et al.[26] (TRACE-III trial 2024)	Phase 3, multicenter, prospective, open-label, randomized, blinded-outcome assessment	4.5–24	• TNK 0.25 mg/kg • Standard medical treatment	• TNK 264 • Standard medical treatment 252	Treatment with TNK resulted in a higher percentage of patients with absence of disability (mRS 0–1) at 90 days than standard medical treatment (33.0% vs. 24.2%; relative rate 1.37; 95% CI; 1.04–1.81; $p = 0.03$)

(EVT: endovascular therapy; mRS: modified Rankin scale; PROBE: prospective randomized open label, blinded–endpoint trial)

Time Window up to 4.5 Hours

Alteplase-Tenecteplase Trial Evaluation for stroke Thrombolysis (ATTEST) and Norwegian Tenecteplase stroke Trial (NOR-TEST) both used only CT scan for enrolling the patients and window period was <4.5 hours.[20,21] Both showed no difference between TNK and alteplase with respect to efficacy and safety outcome.

A meta-analysis by Thelengana et al. in 2018, included 1,334 patients from four RCTs.[27] There were no significant differences between TNK and alteplase with respect to excellent and good functional outcome at 90 days, however, TNK group had significantly better early major neurological improvement [RR = 1.56, 95 CI (1.00, 2.43), $p = 0.05$].

The TNK versus alteplase before endovascular therapy (EVT) for ischemic stroke (EXTEND-1A) randomized patients with large vessel occlusion (LVO) eligible for mechanical thrombectomy between rtPA/TNK (0.25 mg/kg) within 4.5 hours of stroke onset.[22] It was an open label blinded endpoint noninferiority randomized trial. It showed higher incidence of reperfusion (22% vs. 10%, $p = 0.03$) and better functional outcome in TNK group as compared to rtPA group. EXTEND-IA TNK part 2 was done to compare 0.4 mg/kg versus 0.25 mg/kg dose of TNK for improvement of reperfusion before EVT in LVO ischemic stroke.[23] Dose of 0.4 mg/kg did not significantly improve cerebral reperfusion as compared to 0.25 mg/kg dose of TNK prior to EVT.

NORTEST trial showed that 0.4 mg/Kg TNK has similar efficacy and safety outcome as compared to rtPA for minor stroke.[21] NORTEST 2 part A was a noninferiority open label trial to compare TNK 0.4 mg and rtPA within 4.5 hours window for major stroke having NIHSS score > 6.[28] However, the trial was prematurely terminated as TNK dose of 0.4 mg/kg resulted in worse safety and functional outcome compared to alteplase. Any ICH was significantly more frequent with TNK (21%) than with alteplase (7%) of 104 patients [unadjusted OR 3.68 (CI 1.24–10.21), $p = 0.013$].

In Act Trial, 1600 patient were enrolled and randomized to TNK (0.25 mg/Kg) and rtPA (0.9 mg/kg) for acute ischemic stroke within time window of <4.5 hours.[24] 296 (36.9%) of patients in TNK and 266 (34.8%) of 765 patient in alteplase group had mRS score of 0-1 at 90-120 days. [unadjusted RD 2.1%, 95% CI (2.6–6.9)] meeting the prespecified noninferiority threshold.

Time Window up to 6 Hours

Parsons et al.[19] randomized 75 patients to receive alteplase (0.9 mg/kg) or TNK (0.1 mg/kg) < 6 hours after the onset of ischemic stroke in a phase 2B prospective randomized open label, blinded endpoint trial. The eligibility criteria were a perfusion lesion at least 20% greater than the infarct core on computed tomography (CT) perfusion imaging at baseline and an associated vessel occlusion on CT angiography. TNK groups had greater reperfusion ($p = 0.004$) and clinical improvement ($p < 0.001$) at 24 hours than the alteplase group. The higher dose of TNK (0.25 mg/kg) was superior to the lower dose and to alteplase for all efficacy outcomes.

Time Window up to 24 Hours

In TIMELESS trial,[25] patients of acute ischemic stroke with time window of 4.5–24 hours were randomized to TNK (0.25 mg/kg) and placebo. Patients had to have salvageable tissue on perfusion imaging. It did not result in better clinical outcome as compared to placebo. However, nearly 75% of patients underwent thrombectomy in both arms, thus overshadowing any benefit that could have accrued in absence of thrombectomy. Incidence of sICH was similar in two groups, thus establishing the safety of using TNK up to 24 hours.

TRACE-III trial[26] recruited patients of LVO who did not have access to EVT and were randomized to receive TNK (0.25 mg/kg) versus standard medical treatment. The eligibility criteria included patients to have salvageable brain tissue based on CT or magnetic resonance imaging (MRI) perfusion and time window was 4.5–24 hours after the patient was last known to be well. A total of 516 patients were enrolled. The primary outcome was the absence of disability, which was defined as mRS score of 0 or 1 at 90 days. Treatment with TNK resulted in a higher percentage of patients with absence of disability at 90 days than standard medical treatment (33.0% vs. 24.2%; relative rate 1.37; 95% CI 1.04–1.81; $p = 0.03$).

Pairwise Meta-analyses on Safety and Efficacy of Tenecteplase as Compared to Alteplase

Two meta-analyses[6,29] of five randomized trials have demonstrated that TNK and alteplase administered within 4.5 hours of onset have similar efficacy and safety in terms of significant disability or death (mRS 2–6; **Fig. 2**); sICH **(Fig. 3)** and mortality **(Fig. 4)**.

Dose of Tenecteplase

Most of the trials have used a dose of 0.25 mg/kg (maximum 25 mg) and a network

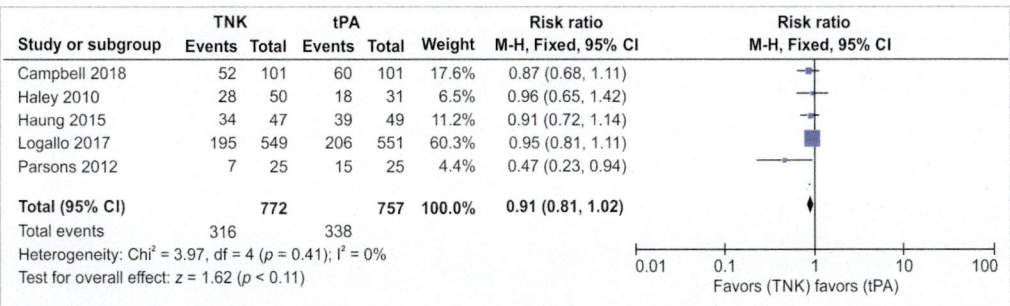

FIG. 2: Outcome: Significant disability (mRS 2–6), comparison TNK versus rtPA.

(mRS: modified Rankin scale; rtPA: recombinant tissue plasminogen activator; TNK: tenecteplase)

meta-analysis[30] has also shown that this dose is the optimum for thrombolysis in acute ischemic stroke. Further, in a systematic review and metanalysis by Rose et al.,[31] 7,913 patients from 26 studies were included to determine the risk of treatment complications between patients treated with TNK and rtPA for acute ischemic stroke. The relative risk of sICH in patients treated with TNK compared with alteplase in 16 studies was 0.89 [95% CI 0.65–1.23); I^2 = 0%]. Among patients treated with low dose (<0.2 mg/kg; four studies), medium dose (0.2–0.39 mg/kg; 13 studies) and high dose (≥ 0.4 mg/kg; three studies) of TNK, the relative risks of symptomatic intracranial hemorrhage were 0.78 [(95% CI 0.22–2.82); I^2 = 0%], 0.77 [(95% CI 0.53–1.14); I^2 = 0%], and 2.31 [(95% CI 0.69–7.75); I^2 = 40%], respectively. It concluded that the risk of complications were comparable when TNK was given in low and medium dose. Thus the dose of TNK recommended for IVT is 0.25 mg/kg (maximum 25 mg).

Treatment with TNK as compared to alteplase was found cost-effective for all acute ischemic patients (including patients with LVO).[32] In a study, patients of acute ischemic stroke with LVO considered for mechanical thrombectomy who received intravenous thrombolytics were retrospectively reviewed.[33] Spontaneous recanalization was significantly more frequently observed in the TNK than in the rtPA groups (unmatched: 23.5% vs. 10.3%, p = 0.032). sICH, 90-day mortality, and functional outcomes were similar. This experience from a real-world

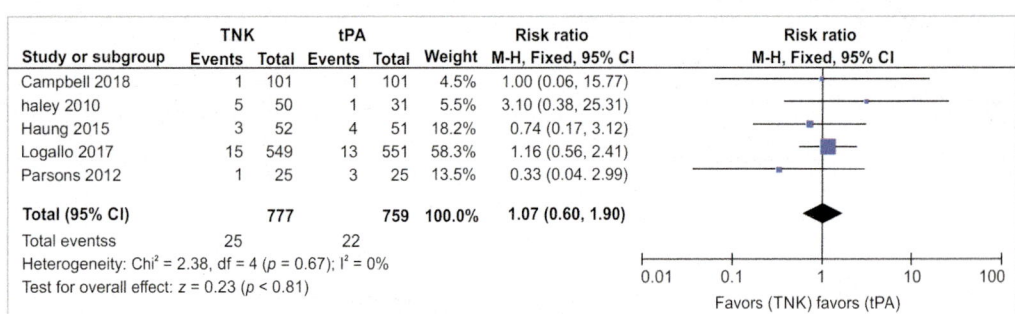

FIG. 3: Outcome: Symptomatic ICH, comparison TNK versus rtPA.
(ICH: intracranial hemorrhage; rtPA: recombinant tissue plasminogen activator; TNK: tenecteplase)

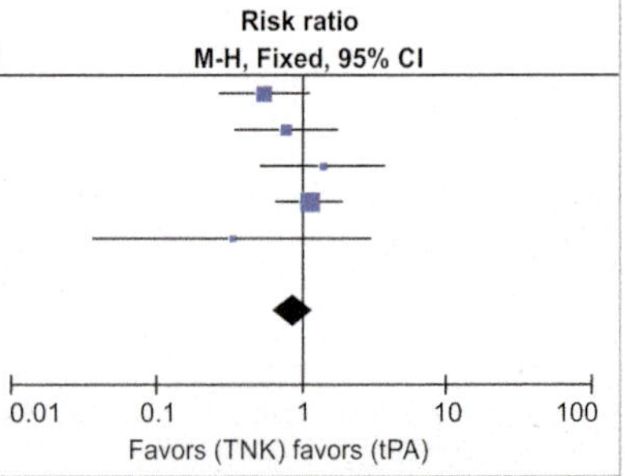

FIG. 4: Outcome: Mortality, comparison TNK versus rtPA.
(rtPA: recombinant tissue plasminogen activator; TNK: tenecteplase)

setting demonstrates superiority of TNK over alteplase; however, there is no evidence from RCT supporting superiority of TNK over alteplase.

OTHER THROMBOLYTIC AGENT

Ideal thrombolytic agent should be effective, has rapid onset of action, has longer half-life, and should be more fibrin specific with less side effects profile particularly bleeding. Streptokinase was studied but resulted in increase in mortality due to increased sICH as compared to placebo.[34] Reteplase has been developed from alteplase and is less fibrin specific than alteplase but has a longer half-life (18 minutes) that allows for double-bolus IV administration. Recently, reteplase has been used in a RCT for acute ischemic stroke within 4.5 hours as a thrombolytic agent in a bolus dose of 18 mg followed by a second bolus of 18 mg as compared to alteplase.[35] About 707 patients were randomized to receive reteplase and 705 to alteplase group. An excellent functional outcome occurred in 79.5% of the patients in the reteplase group and in 70.4% of those in the alteplase group (RR 1.13; 95% CI 1.05–1.21; $p < 0.001$ for noninferiority and $p = 0.002$ for superiority). However, any intracranial hemorrhage at 90 days was higher with reteplase than with alteplase (7.7% vs. 4.9%; RR 1.59; 95% CI 1.00–2.51].

BRIDGING THERAPY

The advantage of bridging thrombolytic treatment with rtPA or TNK before EVT in case of LVO stroke is not clear. On one hand, thrombolytic treatment before EVT may lead to early reperfusion and dissolution of distal residual clots after EVT, on the other hand, prior thrombolysis may make EVT procedure difficult due to fragmentation and distal migration of clot, increased risk of intracranial bleed and delay in start of EVT causing loss of precious time. Many RCT have tried to answer this question: DIRECT MT, DEVT, SKIP, MR CLEAN NO IV, DIRECT SAFE, SWIFT DIRECT **(Table 2)**.[36-41]

TABLE 2: RCTs comparing direct endovascular therapy (dEVT) with bridging therapy.

Trial	Design	Comparison	Patient number	Results
Yang et al.[36] (DIRECT MT 2020)	Multicenter PROBE. Noninferiority, mRS shift noninferiority margin OR 0.80	dEVT vs. BT (with alteplase)	• dEVT (327) • BT (329)	dEVT was noninferior to BT for mRS score at 90 days (Adjusted OR 1.07; 95% CI 0.81–1.40; $p = 0.04$) for noninferiority
Zi et al.[37] (DEVT 2021)	Multicenter PROBE Noninferiority, mRS 0–2 noninferiority margin of 10%	dEVT vs. BT (with alteplase)	• dEVT (116) • BT (118)	Noninferiority of dEVT (54.3%) as compared to BT (46.6%) for functional independence (mRS 0–2) at 3 months [adjusted OR 1.48 (0.81–2.74)]
Suzuki et al.[38] (SKIP 2021)	Multicenter PROBE Noninferiority, mRS 0–2 noninferiority margin OR 0.74	dEVT vs. BT (with alteplase)	• dEVT (101) • BT (103)	Failed to show the noninferiority of dEVT than BT for favorable outcome (mRS 0–2) at 90 days (59.4% vs. 57.3%, $p = 0.18$ for noninferiority)

Continued

Continued

Trial	Design	Comparison	Patient number	Results
Treurniet et al.[39] (MR CLEAN NO IV 2021)	Multicenter PROBE noninferiority, mRS shift noninferiority margin OR 0.80	dEVT vs. BT (with alteplase)	• dEVT (273) • BT (266)	dEVT neither superior nor inferior to BT for disability outcome at 3 months (adjusted OR 0.84; 95% CI 0.62–1.15; $p = 0.28$)
Mitchell et al.[40] (DIRECT SAFE 2022)	Multicenter PROBE noninferiority trial	dEVT vs. BT (with TNK or alteplase)	• dEVT (148) • BT (147)	Functional independence in 80 (55%) of 146 patients in dEVT group and 89 (61%) of 147 patients in BT group (RD –0.051; 95% CI 0.160–0.059)
Fischer et al.[41] (SWIFT DIRECT 2022)	Multicenter PROBE Noninferiority trial	dEVT vs. BT (with alteplase)	• dEVT (201) • BT (207)	Primary outcome (mRS 0–2 at 90 days) was reached by 114 (57%) of 201 patients assigned to thrombectomy alone and 135 (65%) of 207 patients assigned to intravenous alteplase plus thrombectomy (adjusted RD –7.3%; 95% CI –16.6 to 2.1, lower limit of one-sided 95% CI –15.1%, crossing the noninferiority margin of –12%)

[BT: bridging therapy; dEVT: direct endovascular therapy; mRS: modified Rankin scale; PROBE: prospective randomized open label, blinded–endpoint trial; (alteplase or TNK Before EVT)]

There have been many meta-analyses[42,43] of these RCTs, but the assessment of the level of certainty of evidence have been different. The difference results from nonapplication or inappropriate application of GRADE. According to our meta-analysis,[43] low certainty evidence suggests that, compared with EVT and intravenous alteplase, there is possibly a small decrease in the proportion of patients independent with EVT alone [RR 0.97, 95% CI 0.89–1.05; risk difference (RD) –1.5%; 95% CI –5.4 to 2.5], possibly a small increase in mortality with EVT alone (RR 1.07; 95% CI 0.88–1.29; RD 1.2%; 95% CI –2.0 to 4.9). Moderate certainty evidence suggests that there is probably a small decrease in sICH with EVT alone (RR 0.75; 95% CI 0.52–1.07; RD –1.0%; 95% CI –1.8 to 0.27). However, none of the outcomes show statistically significant difference.

In spite of lack of significant difference in clinically important outcomes, many guidelines have strongly recommended use of bridging thrombolysis. This is probably based on the surrogate outcome of early recanalization. However, given the incremental cost of the thrombolytic agent, IAN-endorsed clinical practice guideline[44] favored direct thrombectomy whenever both options are readily available. However, in settings where EVT is not available or a delay is expected in thrombectomy, bridging with IVT is recommended. It is worth noting that most of the bridging trials have used alteplase as the thrombolytic agent. If a superior thrombolytic agent becomes established in terms of safety and efficacy, then bridging trials may yield different results.

MODIFICATIONS IN SELECTION CRITERIA OF INTRAVENOUS THROMBOLYSIS THERAPY

Age

Meta-analysis by Bluhmki et al.[45] evaluated patient data from seven RCT and concluded that IVT has a positive benefit risk profile among patient age > 80 year. Though old age is associated with poor outcomes and increased risk of sICH, IVT within 3 hours of window is recommended for patient < 80 and >80 years of age.[46]

Minor Stroke

The PRISMS RCT[47] randomized 156 patients to IV alteplase and 157 patients to oral aspirin 325 mg with placebo in patient of low NIHSS score (0–5) having nondisabling deficits. Alteplase did not increase the likelihood of good functional outcome at 90 days (78.2% vs. 81.5%, adjusted RD –1.1%; 95% CI –9.4 to 7.3). American Heart Association (AHA) guidelines 2019 update[48] added new recommendation that "for otherwise eligible patients with mild nondisabling stroke symptoms (NIHSS score 0–5), IV alteplase is not recommended for patients who could be treated within 3 or 4.5 hours of ischemic stroke symptom onset or patient last known well or at baseline state".

RAPIDLY IMPROVING SYMPTOMS

The NINDS trial excluded patients with rapidly improving symptoms for IVT presenting within 3 hours. The rationale was not to give alteplase in patients of transient ischemic attack who were recovering rapidly. 2013 AHA/American Stroke Association (ASA) guidelines[49] also mention this as a relative contraindication. However, in many cases transient improvements can plateau after some time resulting in significant residual deficits. AHA guidelines 2019 update[48] has recommended alteplase treatment in patients who present with moderate-to-severe ischemic stroke but likely to remain moderately impaired and potentially disabled in the judgement of examiner. Delaying treatment with alteplase to monitor for further improvement is not recommended.

Cerebral Microbleeds

Risk of sICH in patients with >10 cortical microbleeds is greater than in those with no cerebral microbleeds (CMBs) (1–4.4%).[50] Meta-analysis of four studies concluded that the presence of CMBs was associated with worse outcomes after IV alteplase compared with patients without CMBs [OR 1.58 (95% CI 1.18–2.14); $p = 0.002$].[51] However, it is not clear whether these adverse effects due to CMBs fully negate the benefits of alteplase. AHA guidelines 2019 update recommended that treatment with IVT may be reasonable if there is potential for substantial benefit in patients who have high burden of CMBs (>10) on previous brain MRI.

CONCLUSION

The time window for IVT is not limited to 4.5 hours and can be extended up to 24 hours with the help of advanced imaging. MRI brain can also guide IVT in wake up stroke patients with unknown time of onset of stroke. TIMELESS trial has established the safety of TNK up to 24 hours of onset of ischemic stroke. TRACE-III trial showed effectiveness of TNK in Chinese population as compared to standard medical treatment with time window from 4.5 to 24 hours in group of patients who did not have access to EVT; however, further trials for time window between 4.5 and 24 hours are needed to establish the efficacy of TNK in this group of patients.

The TNK has many advantages like bolus injection, less cost, probably higher rates of recanalization in LVO ischemic stroke and comparable risk of complications as compared to alteplase. At present, there is enough evidence to prove noninferiority of TNK over alteplase for acute ischemic stroke and even evidence of superiority in some prospective observational studies. However, further RCT are needed to prove superiority of TNK over alteplase. It has begun to replace alteplase as IVT of choice because of above advantages in several settings including Canada.

For patients with LVO ischemic stroke, direct EVT is likely noninferior to bridging therapy. However, further trials with use of TNK as bridging therapy are needed to confirm this.

Many of the exclusion criteria for IVT which were there at the time of NINDS trial have been modified and permit IVT for patients in window period.

Use of newer thrombolytics such as reteplase has resulted in better outcome; however further studies are needed to confirm the safety and efficacy as compared to currently established thrombolytic agents, TNK, and alteplase.

REFERENCES

1. Kamalakannan S, Gudlavalleti ASV, Gudlavalleti VSM, Goenka S, Kuper H. Incidence & prevalence of stroke in India: A systematic review. Indian J Med Res. 2017;146(2):175-85.
2. The National Institute of Neurological Disorders and Stroke rt-PA Stroke Study Group. Tissue plasminogen activator for acute ischemic stroke. N Engl J Med. 1995;333:1581-7.
3. Hacke W, Kaste M, Fieschi C, Toni D, Lesaffre E, von Kummer R, et al. Intravenous thrombolysis with recombinant tissue plasminogen activator for acute hemispheric stroke. The European Cooperative Acute Stroke Study (ECASS). JAMA. 1995;274(13):1017-25.
4. Hacke W, Kaste M, Fieschi C, von Kummer R, Davalos A, Meier D, et al. Randomised double-blind placebo-controlled trial of thrombolytic therapy with intravenous alteplase in acute ischaemic stroke (ECASS II). Second European-Australasian Acute Stroke Study Investigators. Lancet Lond Engl. 1998;352(9136):1245-51.
5. Emberson J, Lees KR, Lyden P, Blackwell L, Albers G, Bluhmki E, et al; Stroke Thrombolysis Trialists' Collaborative Group. Effect of treatment delay, age, and stroke severity on the effects of intravenous thrombolysis with alteplase for acute ischaemic stroke: A meta-analysis of individual patient data from randomised trials. Lancet. 2014;384(9958):1929-35.
6. Prasad K, Kumar A, Pandit AK. Evidence for Thrombolytic Therapies in Acute Ischemic Stroke: A New Look. Reviews in Neurology, Stroke. India: Wolters Kluwer (India) Pvt. Ltd; 2019. pp. 207-9.
7. Wardlaw JM, Murray V, Berge E, del Zoppo GJ. Thrombolysis for acute ischaemic stroke. Cochrane Database Syst Rev. 2014;2014(7):CD000213.
8. Clark WM, Wissman S, Albers GW, Jhamandas JH, Madden KP, Hamilton S. Recombinant tissue-type plasminogen activator (Alteplase) for ischemic stroke 3 to 5 hours after symptom onset. The ATLANTIS Study: A randomized controlled trial. Alteplase Thrombolysis for Acute Noninterventional Therapy in Ischemic Stroke. JAMA. 1999;282(21):2019-26.
9. Hacke W, Kaste M, Bluhmki E, Brozman M, Dávalos A, Guidetti D, et al. Thrombolysis with alteplase 3 to 4.5 hours after acute ischemic stroke. N Engl J Med. 2008;359:1317-29.
10. Alper BS, Foster G, Thabane L, Rae-Grant A, Malone-Moses M, Manheimer E. Thrombolysis with alteplase 3-4.5 hours after acute ischaemic stroke: trial reanalysis adjusted for baseline imbalances. BMJ Evid Based Med. 2020;25(5):168-71.
11. Emberson J, Lees KR, Lyden P, Blackwell L, Albers G, Bluhmki E, et al; Stroke Thrombolysis Trialists' Collaborative Group. Effect of treatment delay, age, and stroke severity on the effects of intravenous thrombolysis with alteplase for acute ischaemic stroke: a meta-analysis of individual patient data from randomised trials. Lancet. 2014;384(9958):1929-35.
12. Ma H, Campbell BCV, Parsons MW, Churilov L, Levi CR, Hsu C, et al. Thrombolysis guided by perfusion imaging up to 9 hours after onset of stroke. N Engl J Med. 2019;380:1795-803.

13. Davis SM, Donnan GA, Parsons MW, Levi C, Butcher KS, Peeters A, et al. Effects of alteplase beyond 3 h after stroke in the Echoplanar Imaging Thrombolytic Evaluation Trial (EPITHET): a placebo-controlled randomised trial. Lancet Neurol. 2008;7:299-309.
14. Ringleb P, Bendszus M, Bluhmki E, Donnan G, Eschenfelder C, Fatar M, et al. Extending the time window for intravenous thrombolysis in acute ischemic stroke using magnetic resonance imaging-based patient selection. Int J Stroke. 2019;14:483-90.
15. Campbell BCV, Ma H, Ringleb PA, Parsons MW, Churilov L, Bendszus M, et al. Extending thrombolysis to 4.5-9 h and wake-up stroke using perfusion imaging: a systematic review and meta-analysis of individual patient data. Lancet. 2019;394:139-47.
16. Smalling RW. Molecular biology of plasminogen activators: what are the clinical implications of drug design? Am J Cardiol. 1996;78:2-7.
17. Assessment of the Safety and Efficacy of a New Thrombolytic (ASSENT-2) Investigators; Van De Werf F, Adgey J, Ardissino D, Armstrong PW, Aylward P, Barbash G, et al. Single-bolus tenecteplase compared with front-loaded alteplase in acute myocardial infarction: the ASSENT-2 double-blind randomised trial. Lancet. 1999;354:716-22
18. Haley EC Jr, Lyden PD, Johnston KC, Hemmen TM; TNK in Stroke Investigators. A pilot dose-escalation safety study of tenecteplase in acute ischemic stroke. Stroke. 2005;36:607-12.
19. Parsons M, Spratt N, Bivard A, Campbell B, Chung K, Miteff F, et al. A randomized trial of tenecteplase versus alteplase for acute ischemic stroke. N Engl J Med. 2012;366:1099-107.
20. Huang X, Cheripelli BK, Lloyd SM, Kalladka D, Moreton FC, Siddiqui A, et al. Alteplase versus tenecteplase for thrombolysis after ischaemic stroke (ATTEST): a phase 2, randomised, open-label, blinded endpoint study. Lancet Neurol. 2015;14:368-76.
21. Logallo N, Novotny V, Assmus J, Kvistad CE, Alteheld L, Rønning OM, et al. Tenecteplase versus alteplase for management of acute ischaemic stroke (NOR-TEST): a phase 3, randomised, open-label, blinded endpoint trial. Lancet Neurol. 2017;16:781-8.
22. Campbell BCV, Mitchell PJ, Churilov L, Yassi N, Kleinig TJ, Dowling RJ, et al. Tenecteplase versus alteplase before thrombectomy for ischemic stroke. N Engl J Med. 2018;378:1573-82.
23. Campbell BCV, Mitchell PJ, Churilov L, Yassi N, Kleinig TJ, Dowling RJ, et al. Effect of intravenous tenecteplase dose on cerebral reperfusion before thrombectomy in patients with large Vessel occlusion ischemic stroke: the EXTEND-IA TNK part 2 randomized clinical trial. JAMA. 2020;323:1257-65.
24. Menon BK, Buck BH, Singh N, Deschaintre Y, Almekhlafi MA, Coutts SB, et al; AcT Trial Investigators. Intravenous tenecteplase compared with alteplase for acute ischaemic stroke in Canada (AcT): A pragmatic, multicentre, open-label, registry-linked, randomised, controlled, non-inferiority trial. Lancet. 2022;400(10347):161-9.
25. Albers GW, Jumaa M, Purdon B, Zaidi SF, Streib C, Shuaib A, et al; TIMELESS Investigators. Tenecteplase for Stroke at 4.5 to 24 Hours with Perfusion-Imaging Selection. N Engl J Med. 2024;390(8):701-11.
26. Xiong Y, Campbell BCV, Schwamm LH, Meng X, Jin A, Parsons MW, et al; TRACE-III Investigators. Tenecteplase for Ischemic Stroke at 4.5 to 24 Hours without Thrombectomy. N Engl J Med. 2024;391(3):203-12.
27. Thelengana A, Radhakrishnan DM, Prasad M, Kumar A, Prasad K. Tenecteplase versus alteplase in acute ischemic stroke: Systematic review and meta-analysis. Acta Neurol Belg. 2019;119(3):359-67.
28. Kvistad CE, Næss H, Helleberg BH, Idicula T, Hagberg G, Nordby LM, et al. Tenecteplase versus alteplase for the management of acute ischaemic stroke in Norway (NOR-TEST 2, part A): A phase 3, randomised, open-label, blinded endpoint, non-inferiority trial. Lancet Neurol. 2022;21(6):511-9.
29. Burgos AM, Saver JL. Evidence that Tenecteplase Is Noninferior to Alteplase for Acute Ischemic Stroke: Meta-Analysis of 5 Randomized Trials. Stroke. 2019;50(8):2156-62.
30. Srisurapanont K, Uawithya E, Dhanasomboon P, Pollasen N, Thiankhaw K. Comparative efficacy and safety among different doses of tenecteplase for acute ischemic stroke: A systematic review and network meta-analysis. J Stroke Cerebrovasc Dis. 2024;33(8):107822.
31. Rose D, Cavalier A, Kam W, Cantrell S, Lusk J, Schrag M, et al. Complications of Intravenous Tenecteplase Versus Alteplase for the Treatment of Acute Ischemic Stroke: A Systematic Review and Meta-Analysis. Stroke. 2023;54(5):1192-204.
32. Nguyen CP, Lahr MM, van der Zee DJ, van Voorst H, Roos YB, Uyttenboogaart M, et al. Cost-effectiveness of tenecteplase versus alteplase for acute ischemic stroke. Eur Stroke J. 2023;8(3):638-46.

33. Hendrix P, Collins MK, Griessenauer CJ, Goren O, Melamed I, Weiner GM, et al. Tenecteplase versus alteplase before mechanical thrombectomy: experience from a US healthcare system undergoing a system-wide transition of primary thrombolytic. J Neurointerv Surg. 2023;15(e2):e277-81.
34. Multicenter Acute Stroke Trial--Europe Study Group, Hommel M, Cornu C, Boutitie F, Boissel JP. Thrombolytic therapy with streptokinase in acute ischemic stroke. N Engl J Med. 1996;335:145-50.
35. Li S, Gu HQ, Li H, Wang X, Jin A, Guo S, et al; RAISE Investigators. Reteplase versus Alteplase for Acute Ischemic Stroke. N Engl J Med. 2024;390(24):2264-73.
36. Yang P, Zhang Y, Zhang L, Zhang Y, Treurniet KM, Chen W, et al. Endovascular thrombectomy with or without intravenous alteplase in acute stroke. N Engl J Med. 2020;382:1981-93.
37. Zi W, Qiu Z, Li F, Sang H, Wu D, Luo W, et al. Effect of endovascular treatment alone vs intravenous alteplase plus endovascular treatment on functional independence in patients with acute ischemic stroke: the DEVT randomized clinical trial. JAMA. 2021;325:234-43.
38. Suzuki K, Matsumaru Y, Takeuchi M, Morimoto M, Kanazawa R, Takayama Y, et al. Effect of mechanical thrombectomy without vs with intravenous thrombolysis on functional outcome among patients with acute ischemic stroke: the SKIP randomized clinical trial. JAMA. 2021;325:244-53.
39. Treurniet KM, LeCouffe NE, Kappelhof M, Emmer BJ, van Es ACGM, Boiten J, et al; MR CLEAN-NO IV Investigators. MR CLEAN-NO IV: intravenous treatment followed by endovascular treatment versus direct endovascular treatment for acute ischemic stroke caused by a proximal intracranial occlusion-study protocol for a randomized clinical trial. Trials. 2021;22(1):141.
40. Mitchell PJ, Yan B, Churilov L, Dowling RJ, Bush SJ, Bivard A, et al; DIRECT-SAFE Investigators. Endovascular thrombectomy versus standard bridging thrombolytic with endovascular thrombectomy within 4·5 h of stroke onset: an open-label, blinded-endpoint, randomised non-inferiority trial. Lancet. 2022;400(10346):116-25.
41. Fischer U, Kaesmacher J, Strbian D, Eker O, Cognard C, Plattner PS, et al. SWIFT DIRECT Collaborators. Thrombectomy alone versus intravenous alteplase plus thrombectomy in patients with stroke: an open-label, blinded-outcome, randomised non-inferiority trial. Lancet. 2022;400(10346):104-15.
42. Katsanos AH, Turc G, Psychogios M, Kaesmacher J, Palaiodimou L, Stefanou MI, et al. Utility of Intravenous Alteplase Prior to Endovascular Stroke Treatment: A Systematic Review and Meta-analysis of RCTs. Neurology. 2021;97(8):e777-84.
43. Wang X, Ye Z, Busse JW, Hill MD, Hill MD, Smith EE, Guyatt GH, et al. Endovascular thrombectomy with or without intravenous alteplase for acute ischemic stroke due to large vessel occlusion: a systematic review and meta-analysis of randomized trials. Stroke Vasc Neurol. 2022;7(6):510-7.
44. Ye Z, Busse JW, Hill MD, Lindsay MP, Lindsay MP, Guyatt GH, Prasad K, et al. Endovascular thrombectomy and intravenous alteplase in patients with acute ischemic stroke due to large vessel occlusion: A clinical practice guideline. J Evid Based Med. 2022;15(3):263-71.
45. Bluhmki E, Danays T, Biegert G, Hacke W, Lees KR. Alteplase for acute ischemic stroke in patients aged >80 years: pooled analyses of individual patient data. Stroke. 2020;51:2322-31.
46. Demaerschalk BM, Kleindorfer DO, Adeoye OM, Demchuk AM, Fugate JE, Grotta JC, et al; American Heart Association Stroke Council and Council on Epidemiology and Prevention. Scientific Rationale for the Inclusion and Exclusion Criteria for Intravenous Alteplase in Acute Ischemic Stroke: A Statement for Healthcare Professionals From the American Heart Association/American Stroke Association. Stroke. 2016;47(2):581-641.
47. Khatri P, Kleindorfer DO, Devlin T, Sawyer RN Jr, Starr M, Mejilla J, et al; PRISMS Investigators. Effect of Alteplase vs Aspirin on Functional Outcome for Patients With Acute Ischemic Stroke and Minor Nondisabling Neurologic Deficits: The PRISMS Randomized Clinical Trial. JAMA. 2018;320(2):156-66.
48. Powers WJ, Rabinstein AA, Ackerson T, Adeoye OM, Bambakidis NC, Becker K, et al. Guidelines for the Early Management of Patients With Acute Ischemic Stroke: 2019 Update to the 2018 Guidelines for the Early Management of Acute Ischemic Stroke: A Guideline for Healthcare Professionals From the American Heart Association/American Stroke Association. Stroke. 2019;50(12):e344-e418.
49. Jauch EC, Saver JL, Adams HP Jr, et al; American Heart Association Stroke Council; Council on Cardiovascular Nursing; Council on Peripheral Vascular Disease; Council on Clinical Cardiology. Guidelines for the early management of patients with acute ischemic stroke: a guideline for

healthcare professionals from the American Heart Association/American Stroke Association. Stroke. 2013;44(3):870-947.

50. Tsivgoulis G, Zand R, Katsanos AH, Turc G, Nolte CH, Jung S, et al. Risk of symptomatic intracerebral hemorrhage after intravenous thrombolysis in patients with acute ischemic stroke and high cerebral microbleed burden: a meta-analysis. JAMA Neurol. 2016;73:675-83.

51. Charidimou A, Shoamanesh A; International META-MICROBLEEDS Initiative. Clinical relevance of microbleeds in acute stroke thrombolysis: comprehensive meta-analysis. Neurology. 2016;87:1534-41.

Artificial Intelligence in Acute Stroke Management

Mohan Leslie Noone

ABSTRACT

Artificial intelligence (AI) is revolutionizing acute stroke management. Deep learning, a subset of machine learning, has been used to learn from data without explicit programming, enabling AI systems to match and even surpass human experts. AI has applications in imaging analysis, such as the Alberta Stroke Program Early CT Score (ASPECTS), large vessel occlusion, perfusion mismatch, collaterals, and hemorrhage detection, with platforms such as Aidoc, Avicenna.AI, Brainomix, Qure.AI, RapidAI, and Viz.AI. AI tools are now available which improve the speed and resolution of imaging. AI has also been used to predict short-term and long-term functional outcomes, such as functional independence, and improve care optimization. Public datasets, such as the Ischemic Stroke Lesion Segmentation (ISLES) challenge, provide pooled and annotated data for AI model development, driving the entire landscape forward. AI is poised to have significant positive impacts on acute stroke care, particularly in imaging, care optimization, documentation, and rehabilitation.

Keywords: Acute stroke, Deep learning, Machine learning, Imaging.

INTRODUCTION

Artificial intelligence (AI) refers to computer systems capable of performing tasks that typically require human intelligence, such as visual perception, speech and language processing, and decision making from complex data. The current boom in AI is largely driven by to machine learning (ML), and its subset, deep learning (DL). ML refers to AI systems which learn from data without explicit programming, using either human-labeled data (supervised learning) or by identifying patterns in unlabeled data (unsupervised learning). Almost all applications in healthcare utilize supervised ML.

Deep learning, a sophisticated form of ML, involves multiple layers of processing nodes (often called neurons), which were initially inspired by biological neurons but function through numerical inputs, batch multiplications, and nonlinear operations. Once trained on sufficient-labeled data, ML systems can surpass human experts by effectively pooling the knowledge of numerous professionals. They operate without fatigue, maintain peak efficiency without breaks, and are easily scalable, making them ideal for delivering high-quality, data-driven, and personalized healthcare. Stroke management is no exception.

BACKGROUND

Searching PubMed for "Artificial Intelligence" and "Acute Stroke" gives around 230 results, excluding reviews, and the breakup is given in **Table 1**.

Thus, beyond image analysis, the main applications of AI in acute stroke include outcome prediction, care optimization, and rehabilitation. Improving the speed and resolution of imaging using AI to extrapolate additional information, using generative approaches, is also an area of active research.

TABLE 1: Category-wise counts of PubMed articles on searching "Artificial Intelligence" and "Acute Stroke".

Category	Count
Imaging–Analysis	66
Outcome prediction	50
Rehabilitation	43
Robotics	29
Imaging: Speed and resolution	14
Care optimization	12
Miscellaneous	16

APPLICATIONS

Imaging—Analysis

Artificial intelligence has found application in the following key areas of acute stroke imaging analysis:
- Alberta Stroke Program Early CT Score (ASPECTS)
- Large vessel occlusion (LVO)
- Perfusion mismatch
- Collaterals
- Hemorrhage detection

Commercially available and approved platforms providing such features include Aidoc, Avicenna.AI, Brainomix, Qure.AI, RapidAI, and Viz.AI.[1]

Evaluation of Performance of AI on Region Mapping Tasks

Tasks such as ASPECTS, collaterals, and perfusion mapping require mapping of areas, and a commonly used statistic to evaluate the performance on such tasks is the Dice similarity coefficient.[2] Dice similarity coefficient is a spatial overlap index and a reproducibility validation metric. It is also called the proportion of specific agreement. Such region marking tasks are commonly called "image segmentation" tasks in AI terminology.

Alberta Stroke Program Early CT Score

The AI systems have been shown to match or even exceed human radiologists at ASPECTS scoring. However, in patients with acute stroke with baseline CT abnormalities, one of the leading vendors, Brainomix e-ASPECTS did not perform as well as neuroradiologists when scoring ASPECTS.[3] Qure.AI reported a Dice similarity coefficient of 0.64 for middle cerebral artery (MCA) anatomy segmentation and 0.72 for infarct segmentation **(Fig. 1)**.[4]

Large Vessel Occlusion Detection

Viz. LVO was the first US Food and Drug Administration (US FDA)-approved AI/ML-enabled technology for stroke.[5] The company reported an area under the receiver operating curve (AUC) of 0.91 and reduced time from scan to notification from 58 to 7 minutes, in data submitted to the US FDA. Other commercially available LVO detection is provided by RapidAI, Brainomix, Qure.AI, and others. As described below, this can be incorporated into a comprehensive stroke management care flow to quickly triage patients for thrombectomy **(Fig. 2)**.

CT and MR Perfusion, Collateral Assessment

The analysis of CT and MR perfusion and collateral assessment to detect viable tissue for intervention can be enhanced by AI/ML by enabling better thresholding and faster

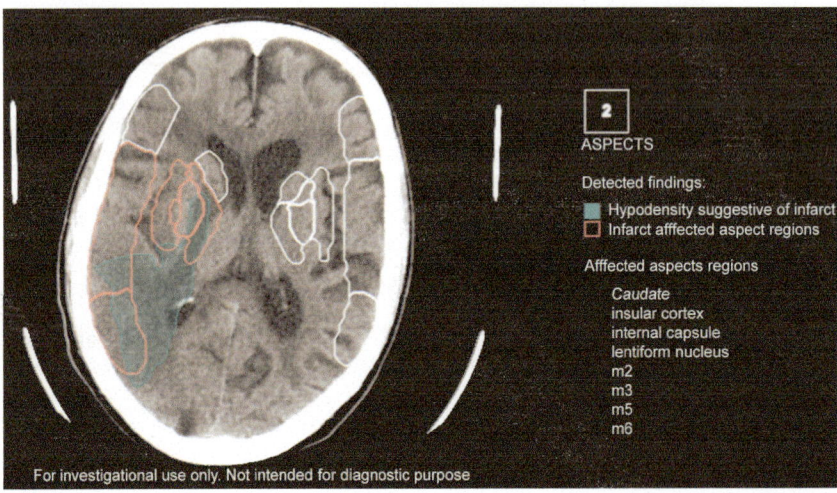

FIG. 1: Alberta Stroke Program Early CT Score (ASPECTS) using artificial intelligence (AI).
Courtesy: Qure.AI.

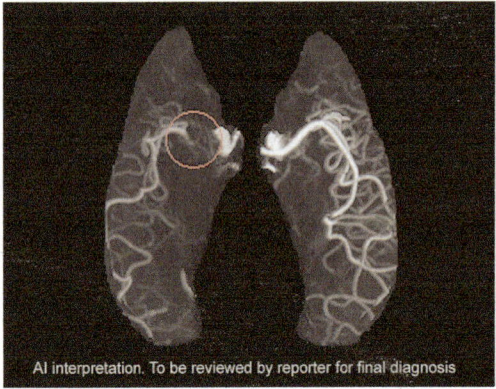

FIG. 2: Large vessel occlusion detection using artificial intelligence (AI).
Courtesy: Qure.AI.

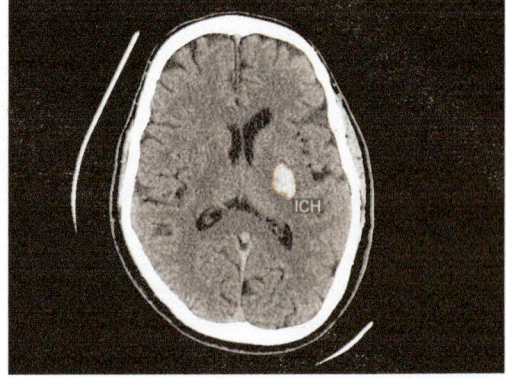

FIG. 3: Intracranial hemorrhage detection using artificial intelligence (AI).
Courtesy: Qure.AI.

processing times. The RapidAI software has been particularly popular in this regard, and it has been used in influential stroke clinical trials around the world.[6]

Intracranial Hemorrhage Identification

BriefCase was the first FDA-approved, AI/ML-enabled technology for the identification of intracranial hemorrhage (ICH) on CT scans. The performance of AI models in ICH identification is typically higher than tasks such as ASPECTS and LVO.[5] Qure.AI reported an AUC of 0.92 for detecting ICH (0.90 for intraparenchymal, 0.96 for intraventricular, 0.92 for subdural, 0.93 for extradural, and 0.90 for subarachnoid) on the Qure25k dataset, which consisted of 21,095 scans **(Fig. 3)**.[7]

Outcome Prediction

Short Term

The AI/ML has been studied in the short-term prediction of imaging biomarkers such as final infarct volume and hemorrhagic transformation, from initial imaging data. Performance has been variable with sensitivity and specificity of 89% and 60% for predicting hemorrhagic transformation using a neural network from initial MRI perfusion and diffusion images.[6]

Long Term

Predicting long-term functional outcome is of importance in stroke treatment and research. Functional independence is generally defined as a modified Ranking Score of 2 or less for this purpose. In 1,383 patients from the MR CLEAN Registry, functional independence could be moderately well predicted using baseline variables only (AUC, 0.77–0.79) but well predicted when treatment variables were included (0.88–0.91).[6] As expected, AI models perform better with more relevant data inputs, specifically for a task like long-term functional outcome which depends on several factors.

Care Optimization

Acute stroke care is highly time bound, with door to needle and door to puncture times as clear targets for optimization. Mobile app-based workflows have been studied and demonstrated to improve and streamline acute stroke care pathways.[8] Incorporating AI-based analytics, and predictions could help to further refine care.[9] AI-based image analysis along with decision support which is based on the current guidelines would enable peripheral centers to rapidly and accurately thrombolyse and triage patients who need referral for thrombectomy (the drip and ship model).

Speed and Quality of Imaging

AI-inspired methods can enhance the quality of medical images, enabling faster acquisition or lower doses. For instance, AI can de-noise MR brain perfusion images using arterial spin labeling, allowing for shorter scan times. Considering the concerns about gadolinium deposition from MR contrast agents, AI techniques that reduce the necessary amount of gadolinium for diagnostic imaging could be beneficial for bolus perfusion-weighted imaging. Convolutional neural networks (CNNs) can also be employed to lower radiation doses, addressing radiation concerns associated with CT perfusion imaging, which is a relatively high-dose procedure.[6]

Deep learning can predict gold standard imaging biomarkers when direct measurement is infeasible. For example, cerebral blood flow (CBF) imaging typically relies on O15-water positron emission tomography, which requires an on-site cyclotron due to the isotope's short half-life, limiting its use in acute stroke cases. A deep CNN can be trained to predict O15-water CBF using MR images from stable patients and then applied in acute settings to estimate true perfusion. This method could be extended to predict CT perfusion results from CT and CT angiography (CTA) images or Tmax lesions from noncontrast MR scans, optimizing imaging in various contexts.[6]

Rehabilitation and Robotics

While not strictly confined to acute stroke, significant work has been done in the application of AI in stroke rehabilitation, including the use of robotics. For instance, two FDA-approved technologies designed to enhance poststroke recovery are BrainQ and IpsiHand. BrainQ is a noninvasive brain–computer interface (BCI) device that uses extremely low-frequency and low-intensity electromagnetic fields (ELF-EMF) to aid poststroke recovery. BrainQ's technology employs ML to analyze motor-related spectral features from electrophysiology measurements and translates them into ELF-EMF treatments, promoting neuroplasticity. In a pilot trial, patients receiving ELF-EMF treatment showed superior recovery without adverse events compared to a control group who received sham treatment. The IpsiHand Upper Extremity Rehabilitation System (IpsiHand) received FDA breakthrough status in April 2021, becoming the first FDA-approved BCI device for motor rehabilitation in poststroke patients which uses an electroencephalogram (EEG) recording headset to translate movement intent from the uninjured brain hemisphere into physical movements of a robotic exoskeleton on the impaired limb. In a study, 10 stroke survivors showed significant arm functionality improvement after 12 weeks of IpsiHand therapy.[5]

Miscellaneous Applications

Prediction of associated coronary artery disease, EEG analysis in stroke, estimation of mechanism of stroke in embolic stroke of unknown source, predicting onset time from imaging, and fall prediction are some other reported applications of AI in acute stroke.

Large Language Models

Large language models (LLMs) such as ChatGPT have access to vast data and knowledge and can perform quite well on medical tasks. Rao et al. studied the accuracy of ChatGPT after inputting 36 published clinical vignettes from the *Merck Sharp & Dohme (MSD) Clinical Manual*. The generated differential diagnoses, diagnostic testing, final diagnosis, and management based on patient age, gender, and case acuity were assessed by human scorers

ChatGPT achieved an overall accuracy of 71.7% across all clinical vignettes. The LLM demonstrated the highest performance in making a final diagnosis with an accuracy of 76.9% and the lowest performance in generating an initial differential diagnosis with an accuracy of 60.3%.[10]

Google's Med-PaLM is a LLM trained specifically on medical knowledge.[11] The second version. Med-PaLM 2 scored 85.4% in USMLE. The LLMs have ushered a new era of high-level language and knowledge-based AI upon the world. The practical applications of LLMs in healthcare, including acute stroke, are still evolving, and may include medical question answering, medical record generation from raw input such as voice transcripts and other sources, and making customized materials for patient counseling, engagement, and education.

Brain–Computer Interfaces

Companies such as Elon Musk's Neuralink are studying BCIs which have now entered human trials,[12] enabling paralyzed patients to use computers with their thoughts. Further refinement of these technology could provide functional restoration for both motor and sensory impairments caused by stroke, potentially including language expression, mobility, vision, and using devices such as mobile phones and computers. The interface uses AI to process and interpret the electrical activity captured by the electrodes from the brain.

■ PUBLIC DATASETS AND OPEN CHALLENGES

Public data tests provide pooled and annotated data and are a key factor in AI model development. Often such datasets form part of challenges such as the ISLES challenge.[13] This enables rapid development of focused technology that drives the entire landscape forward.

ETHICAL CONCERNS AND BIASES

Artificial intelligence systems are prone to acquire biases from training data. Fair and accurate representation of the intended patient demographic in the training data will help to achieve better results. Hence, developing models from local data is important to get the maximum benefit.

Other ethical concerns in AI include unauthorized use of sources such as copyrighted materials, nonconsented patient data for training and development of AI models. Legal frameworks governing such use cases are still evolving. Frameworks such as the Ayushman Bharat Digital Mission incorporate mechanism for default consent for using anonymized and deidentified data for training of AI.

CONCLUSION

Artificial intelligence may be considered as a set of technologies that push the boundaries of what machines can do to assist our efforts toward higher levels of quality, consistency, customization, and reliability. With broad applications in imaging, care optimization, documentation, and rehabilitation, AI is poised to have major positive impacts on stroke care. Concerns of bias and unethical use have to be acknowledged and awareness and appropriate frameworks to keep them in check should be developed by professional bodies and administrations. Awareness of this rapidly evolving field and tools available will be important for all involved in the care of acute stroke patients.

REFERENCES

1. Soun JE, Chow DS, Nagamine M, Takhtawala RS, Filippi CG, Yu W, et al. Artificial intelligence and acute stroke imaging. AJNR Am J Neuroradiol. 2021;42:2-11.
2. Zou KH, Warfield SK, Bharatha A, Tempany CM, Kaus MR, Haker SJ, et al. Statistical validation of image segmentation quality based on a spatial overlap index. Acad Radiol. 2004;11(2):178-89.
3. Guberina N, Dietrich U, Radbruch A, Goebel J, Deuschl C, Ringelstein A, et al. Detection of early infarction signs with machine learning-based diagnosis by means of the Alberta Stroke Program Early CT score (ASPECTS) in the clinical routine. Neuroradiology. 2018;60:889-901.
4. Upadhyay U, Ranjan M, Golla S, Tanamala S, Sreenivas P, Chilamkurthy S, et al. (2022). Deep-ASPECTS: A Segmentation-Assisted Model for Stroke Severity Measurement. [online] Available from https://arxiv.org/abs/2203.03622 [Last accessed August, 2024].
5. Chandrabhatla AS, Kuo EA, Sokolowski JD, Kellogg RT, Park M, Mastorakos P. Artificial intelligence and machine learning in the diagnosis and management of stroke: A Narrative Review of United States Food and Drug Administration-Approved Technologies. J Clin Med. 2023;12:3755.
6. Mouridsen K, Thurner P, Zaharchuk G. Artificial intelligence applications in stroke. Stroke. 2020;51:2573-9
7. Chilamkurthy S, Ghosh R, Tanamala S, Biviji M, Campeau NG, Venugopal VK, et al. Deep learning algorithms for detection of critical findings in head CT study cans: a retrospective study. Lancet. 2018;392:2388-96.
8. Noone ML, Moideen F, Krishna RB, Pradeep Kumar VG, Karadan U, Chellenton J, et al. Mobile app based strategy improves door-to-needle time in the treatment of acute ischemic stroke. J Stroke Cerebrovasc Dis. 2020;29(12):105319.
9. Nagaratnam K, Neuhaus A, Briggs JH, Ford GA, Woodhead ZVJ, Maharjan D, et al. Artificial intelligence-based decision support software to improve the efficacy of acute stroke pathway in the NHS: An observational study. Front Neurol. 2024;14:1329643.

10. Rao A, Pang M, Kim J, Kamineni M, Lie W, Prasad AK, et al. Assessing the Utility of ChatGPT Throughout the Entire Clinical Workflow: Development and Usability Study J Med Internet Res. 2023;25:e48659.
11. Singhal K, Azizi S, Tu T, Mahdavi SS, Wei J, Chung HW, et al. Large language models encode clinical knowledge. Nature. 2023;620:172-80.
12. Zhang Y, Wu M. Human brain extended: Neuralink's brain-computer interface trial starts. MedComm Biomater App. 2024;3:10.
13. Hernandez Petzsche MR, de la Rosa E, Hanning U, Wiest R, Valenzuela W, Reyes M, et al. ISLES 2022: A multi-center magnetic resonance imaging stroke lesion segmentation dataset. Sci Data. 2022; 9:762.

Expanding Indications in Acute Ischemic Stroke Reperfusion and Endovascular Therapy

Ashutosh Mahapatra, Dileep R Yavagal

ABSTRACT

Stroke is the leading cause of death and disability worldwide. The establishment of intravenous thrombolysis (IVT) in 1996 for acute ischemic stroke (AIS) and endovascular therapy (EVT) for large vessel occlusion (AIS) in 2015 was landmark advances in stroke therapy. Since then, a steady stream of positive clinical trials has expanded the patients eligible for both IVT and EVT. Here, we review the evidence for new EVT and IVT indications for AIS and their application in clinical practice. We review the extended time window and low NIHSS for IV thrombolysis and the rapidly increasing populations for EVT application, including patients with a large core, low NIHSS at presentation, posterior circulation LVO, and distal occlusions. We also review innovations in stroke care systems for EVT focused on direct-to-angiosuite and telestroke.

Keywords: Stroke, AIS, EVT, IVT.

■ INTRODUCTION

Stroke is the second leading cause of death and the third leading cause of disability worldwide. A recent study estimated the economic burden as estimated by value of welfare lost due to stroke to be $2059.67 billion or 1.66% of the global GDP. Over the last three decades, the advent of intravenous thrombolysis (IVT) and endovascular therapy has dramatically altered the landscape of acute ischemic stroke (AIS) care throughout the world. Initially, IVT and mechanical thrombectomy (MT) were applied to a small, controlled subset of AIS patients, based on the strict inclusion and exclusion criteria. The large effect size of the benefit seen in EVT studies has suggested that patient populations outside the selected ones in the landmark trials would likely benefit. Also, improved thrombectomy devices, stroke imaging, and pharmacological advances have added to the broadening of indications such as distal vessel occlusions. Although broadened applications have allowed treatment of many more patients, the safety and efficacy of these therapies in certain patient populations still remains to be established, and several ongoing studies are investigating their effectiveness.

■ INTRAVENOUS THROMBOLYSIS

Treatment Window Expansion

Beginning in 1995–1996, with the landmark National Institute of Neurological Disorders and Stroke (NINDS) trial, intravenous tissue plasminogen activator (IV-tPA) found its place as an effective therapy for the treatment of AIS patients with a disabling neurological deficit presenting within a 3-hour time window.[1] Although an important breakthrough, and an effective therapy, the strict time window for administration excluded a large portion of patients, with studies reporting the rates of IV-tPA administration ranging from 3 to 9% of all AIS patients.

In 2008, the subsequent European Cooperative Acute Stroke Study III (ECASS-III) trial demonstrated relative safety and effectiveness of IV-tPA administration in the 3–4.5-hour time window.[2] Even this slightly broadened time window increased rates of IV-tPA administration to nearly 20% of all AIS patients.[2]

As comfort with IV-tPA increased with time and experience, the phenomenon of "wake-up strokes" was recognized, and the utilization of new technology (i.e., perfusion-imaging, hyperacute MRI) was adopted, questions regarding the efficacy of IVT in extended windows arose.

The 2018 WAKE-UP trial demonstrated that treatment with IV-tPA with an unknown time of stroke onset and diffusion-weighted imaging (DWI) and fluid-attenuated inverse recovery (FLAIR) mismatch on magnetic resonance imaging (MRI) significantly improved functional outcomes without a significantly increased risk of death or major bleeding.[3] Given the physiology behind DWI and FLAIR imaging, DWI-FLAIR mismatch suggested that the onset of a patients' stroke was likely within a 4.5-hour range.

The 2019 EXTEND trial further demonstrated that treatment with IV-tPA in patients with "salvageable brain tissue" as detected by automated perfusion imaging in patients presenting in the 4.5–9-hour time window after onset of stroke was associated with benefits in functional outcome, without significantly increased risk of death or hemorrhage.[4]

Special mention should be made of the newer thrombolytic drug, tenecteplase (TNK), which has been recently shown in several randomized clinical trials to achieve higher rates of recanalization and reperfusion when compared to alteplase, without higher risk of bleeding. It has also been touted as a less cumbersome medication to administer, as it requires only a one-time bolus dose, as compared to the bolus plus infusion required with alteplase. This has led to many institutions transitioning to the use of TNK. Several ongoing trials have produced mixed results regarding the effectiveness of TNK in extended time windows.

The 2024 TIMELESS trial failed to demonstrate benefit of TNK therapy initiated 4.5–24 hours after stroke onset in patients with middle cerebral artery (MCA) or internal carotid artery (ICA), most of which underwent concurrent MT. There was, however, no significant increase in the risk of bleeding between the TNK group and the placebo group.[5]

A 2024 Chinese study, TRACE-III, however, did show benefit in treatment of TNK administered 4.5–24 hours after stroke onset in patients who did could not receive EVT due to lack of access, at the tradeoff of an overall higher risk of symptomatic intracranial hemorrhage (sICH) when compared to standard medical treatment (3.0% vs. 0.8%).[6]

These studies suggest that IVT remains a viable option in patients with AIS presenting within 9 hours of symptom onset. Appropriate selection of these patients may require the use of advanced imaging modalities to assess the degree of brain tissue at risk. There may be some benefit in pursuing IVT in patients up to 24 hours after stroke onset in special scenarios, such as when the patient does not have access to EVT. There are several ongoing studies which continue to explore these areas.

Stroke with Low National Institute of Health Stroke Scale

More than half of patients with AIS have minor or mild neurological deficits at presentation. The widespread utilization of IVT after the 1995–1996 NINDS trial also concurrently established the National Institute of Health Stroke Scale (NIHSS) as a validated tool for assessing the severity of neurological symptoms in AIS patients. Typically, severe symptoms have been described as an NIHSS > 6. Though the NINDS trial did not specifically address a NIHSS cutoff, mild strokes, or nondisabling strokes (NIHSS 5 or less) was a relative exclusion criterion.

A criticism of the NIHSS has been its poor validity in assessing posterior circulation stroke symptoms. Symptoms such as severe vertigo, dysmetria, and diplopia are typically not scored, but may be associated with significant discomfort and disability for a particular patient. Additionally, patients may present with AIS symptoms that are mild, but related to large vessel occlusion (LVO) on vascular imaging studies, and in these situations, the risk of subsequent decline in neurological status without any treatment may be significant.

To address some of these concerns, several studies have been conducted to assess the safety and efficacy of treating low-NIHSS strokes with IVT. The two largest studies conducted were the PRISMS and MaRISS studies.

PRISMS (2018) studied the safety and efficacy of IV-tPA administered within 3 hours of symptom onset amongst patients with minor deficits (NIHSS 0–5), otherwise judged as not clearly disabling at presentation.[7] The control arm received IV placebo and oral aspirin. The study showed that treatment with alteplase did not increase the likelihood of favorable functional outcome at 90 days, with overall increase in symptomatic ICH in the alteplase arm.

MaRISS (2021) was a prospective observational study which included patients with AIS or TIA and NIHSS 0-5, presenting within 4.5 hours of symptom onset.[8] It determined that a large proportion of stroke patients presenting initially with low NIHSS have a disabled outcome (37% disabled and 25% nonindependent). Alteplase-treated patients within the study did not influence outcome, but there was a suggestion of efficacy noted within the NIHSS 3–5 subgroup.

Thrombolysis in low NIHSS or minor strokes has remained controversial. An analysis of trends in IVT and EVT for low NIHSS in the United States has suggested that the rates of IVT have decreased, with rates of EVT increasing. EVT in low NIHSS is discussed in a following section.

Endovascular Therapy for Ischemic Stroke

In 2015, five landmark trials (MR CLEAN, SWIFT PRIME, REVASCAT, EXTEND-IA, and ESCAPE) showed the dramatic benefit of EVT in patients suffering from AIS in anterior circulation, presenting within the first 6 hours after presumed symptom onset.[9-13] With number-needed-to-treats (NNTs) of 2–8, EVT forever changed the landscape of AIS care as one of the most efficacious therapies in the history of medicine and surgery. Like IVT, the general lack of access to the therapy, and the relatively strict inclusion criteria for eligibility for EVT, limited the number of patients undergoing MT. Many studies have been conducted since that time to expand the indications for EVT, but several areas remain controversial.

Endovascular Therapy for Low NIHSS

The landmark trials have established EVT as the standard of care in patients presenting with AIS with an NIHSS of 6 or greater.

These trials largely excluded patients with mild deficits or low NIHSS, likely to enhance the chances of showing treatment benefit (especially considering the initial negative trials such as IMS-III). Even with low NIHSS, the symptoms of stroke can be devastating to a patient's overall quality of life. For example, a patient may present with isolated severe expressive aphasia secondary to occlusion of the MCA, but only score 5 on NIHSS examination. Lack of data in this subset of patients has raised controversy.

Many factors must be considered when selecting a patient with low NIHSS for EVT. These include assessment of individual patient symptoms, imaging characteristics, and collateral status.[14] There is also a subset of patients which present with low NIHSS initially, and undergo medical management, with subsequent neurological deterioration. The etiology of this has been suspected to be failure of leptomeningeal collaterals. Eventually these patients may be taken for EVT, albeit in a delayed fashion resulting in the potential of worsened neurological outcomes. One study suggested that this phenomenon occurs in almost 20% of patients presenting initially with low NIHSS and concurrent LVO.[15] No clear indicators of neurological deterioration have been ascertained, but some factors predisposing patients may include prolonged time of presentation from symptom onset, volume status, poorly controlled diabetes, and volume status.

Data is scattered in limited to retrospective case series with small sample sizes and a few meta-analyses performed from the available retrospective series. Currently, both the SVIN and SNIS guidelines recommend EVT in patients with low NIHSS with disabling or worsening symptoms. Two ongoing clinical trials are more definitively investigating the efficacy of low NIHSS EVT–ENDOLOW and MOSTE **(Figs. 1A to D)**.[16]

Distal Medium Vessel Occlusions

Another area of controversy is in the realm of performing EVT in more distal occlusions. The landmark trials limited EVT to first and second-order vessels in the anterior circulation (ICA, ICA-T, M1, M2, and A1). Occlusion of vessels beyond these territories were excluded and data on the safety and feasibility of treating distal medium vessel occlusions (DMVOs) is rather limited. DMVOs have varying definitions in the literature, and multiple collaborations are in the process of standardizing the definition of DMVOs. In general, DMVOs refer to M3-M4, A2-A5, P2-P5, PICA, AICA, and SCAs.[17] These

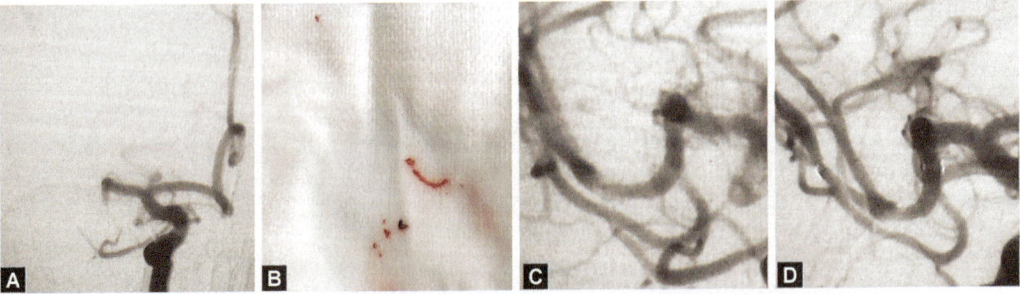

FIGS. 1A TO D: A 57-year-old male presenting with left face, arm, and leg numbness; NIHSS 1. CT angiogram of the brain showed right M1 occlusion. Successful EVT leading to patient being discharged home with NIHSS of 0 on day 3 post-EVT.

(CT: computed tomography; EVT: endovascular therapy; NIHSS: National Institute of Health Stroke Scale)

vessels typically have diameters ranging from 1 to 3 mm.

Based on extrapolations of various population studies, distal and medium vessel occlusions account for approximately 25–40% of all AIS patients. They can occur as primary occlusions and secondary occlusions (from fragmentation of more proximal thrombi because of IVT or EVT), and present as a wide variety of clinical symptoms based on anatomical territories undergoing ischemia.[18]

The rationale for pursuing recanalization of these occlusions with EVT is rather straightforward, as time and time again, revascularization of at-risk territories seems to prove beneficial in essentially all arterial distributions. Additionally, the utility of IVT alone in DMVOs is limited. Although IVT is comparatively more effective for distal occlusions than proximal occlusions, the overall recanalization rates with IVT alone are < 50%, as demonstrated by the INTERRSeCT and PRoveIT studies.[19,20]

There remain, however, reservations from the neurointerventional community. These reservations stem from diagnostic, anatomical, and technical concerns.

Firstly, there are challenges in identifying and diagnosing them in a timely fashion. Although computed tomography angiography (CTA) and magnetic resonance angiography (MRA) provide high reliability in the detection of proximal occlusions, there is decreased spatial resolution due to small caliber of the distal vasculature in DMVOs. Newer imaging technology (wavelet CTA, 7T-MRA) may help in overcoming some of these challenges, but they are of limited availability and significant cost.[18] Currently, a commonly used method of helping identify distal occlusions is CT perfusion (CTP). The ischemic territory is suggested by a wedge-shaped region of hypoperfusion in a typical distal anterior cerebral artery (ACA), MCA, or posterior cerebral artery (PCA) territory.

Distal vessels are overall smaller in diameter when compared to the proximal large vessels. Secondly, as branching occurs, there can be significant anatomic tortuosity affecting these patients, especially those with long-standing history of vascular risk factors. Thirdly, distal vessels tend to be more friable and delicate than their more robust counterparts. The combination of these factors presents significant challenges in catheter/device navigation and the performance of EVT. Most EVT devices have been specifically designed for LVO-targeted EVT. Although smaller size stent-retrievers (SRs) and aspiration catheters have been designed and used successfully, their safety and efficacy have been yet to be studied in large-scale clinical trials.[21]

There is some data to suggest that EVT for DMVOs is comparable in safety profile to EVT for LVOs. The Trevo Retriever Registry subgroup analysis of DMVOs (excluding M2 occlusions), demonstrated similar rates of postprocedure reperfusion, symptomatic ICH, and 90-day-functional outcomes.[22] An analysis of the STAR Registry demonstrates that EVT for DMVO had a higher rate of good outcome (45% vs. 36%, $p = 0.03$), but lower rates of TICI 2b/3 perfusion (78% vs. 84%, $p = 0.04$). A multicenter cohort study with 286 patients with DMVO in the anterior circulation (156 w/EVT, 130 w/medical management) demonstrated no significant differences in clinical outcomes or mortality.[23]

Currently several ongoing randomized controlled trials (RCTs) are working to evaluate the utility of DMVO EVT (DISTALS, DISTAL, ESCAPE-MeVO, DISCOUNT, DUSK) **(Figs. 2A to D)**.[21]

Endovascular Therapy for Posterior Circulation Large Vessel Occlusion

Posterior circulation strokes account for approximately 20% of all strokes. Posterior circulation LVOs are rather

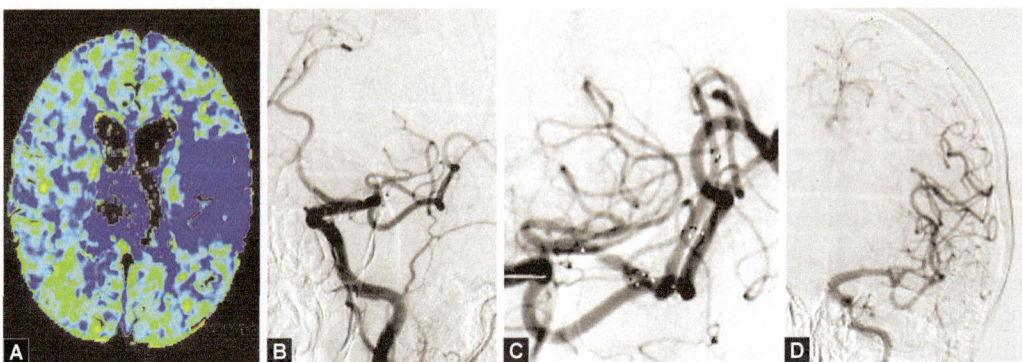

FIGS. 2A TO D: A 79-year-old male presenting with left MCA syndrome with NIHSS of 6 at 2 hours from symptom onset. CTP shows a partial hypoperfusion on MTT map and angio confirms a left mid MCA-M2 segment occlusion. TICI 2c reperfusion post-thrombectomy with stent retriever. Patient discharged at day 4 post-EVT with NIHSS of 1.
(CTP: CT perfusion; EVT: endovascular therapy; MCA: middle cerebral artery; MTT: mean transit time; NIHSS: National Institute of Health Stroke Scale; TICI: thrombolysis in cerebral infarction)

rare, representing approximately 1% of all ischemic strokes (and 5% of LVOs). Given these considerations, posterior circulation LVOs were largely excluded from the initial landmark EVT clinical trials. Certain brands of posterior circulation LVOs, however, are clinically devastating, such as basilar artery occlusions—these can present as a patient with coma, locked-in syndrome, or in extremis/near-death given the effect on the brainstem.[24]

Several recently completed RCTs for posterior circulation EVT (primarily for basilar artery occlusion) have shed some insight into treating these lesions.

The Basilar Artery Occlusion Endovascular Intervention Versus Standard Medical Treatment (BEST) trial enrolled 131 patients (66 in EVT group, 65 in medical management group) within 8 hours of symptoms onset with vertebrobasilar occlusion. This trial was unfortunately plagued by poor recruitment and high crossover rates. There was no difference found in 90-day functional outcomes, mortality, or sICH rates between the two arms, but there was a noted numerically higher rate of sICH in the intervention arm.[25]

The Basilar Artery International Cooperation Study (BASICS) trial enrolled 300 (154 in EVT group and 146 in medical management group) patients, with presentation within 6 hours attributed to a basilar artery occlusion. Again, no significant benefit was found in EVT patients, with similar rates of mortality and sICH.[26]

The Basilar Artery Occlusion Chinese Endovascular (BAOCHE) trial enrolled 217 patients presenting 6–24 hours after symptom onset, randomized to either EVT or medical management. BAOCHE enrolled patients utilizing clinical severity criteria (NIHSS > 5, PC-ASPECTS > 5, and pons midbrain index score of <3). In this study, there was significantly improved outcomes in the EVT arm [Modified Rankin score (mRS) 0–3 in 46% vs. 24%, $p < 0.001$].[27]

The Endovascular Treatment for Acute Basilar Artery Occlusion (ATTENTION) trial, also a Chinese study, enrolled 340 patients presenting within 12 hours of symptom onset, with NIHSS > 10, and PC-ASPECTS of > 5. The chance of achieving a good functional outcome was two times higher in the EVT group (46% vs. 23%, $p < 0.001$).[28]

It is important to note that in both BAOCHE and ATTENTION, several factors contributed to the positive outcomes. Patient selection was stricter in these trials, as they enrolled patients utilizing clinical severity measures and more nuanced imaging criteria. In both studies, there was also a significantly high rate of rescue angioplasty and/or stenting utilized in BAOCHE and ATTENTION (40% and 55%, respectively).

Taken together, the literature and recent trials suggest that EVT for posterior circulation AIS is beneficial, especially in patients with NIHSS > 5 and PC-ASPECTS > 5, who present within 12 hours of symptom onset or last known well. There is less robust benefit in patients presenting in the 12-24-hour window. As with anterior circulation AIS, there is uncertainty of benefit in patients presenting with low NIHSS (<5), beyond 24 hours, or with distal medium vessel posterior circulation occlusions.

Endovascular Therapy for Large Core Acute Ischemic Stroke

The landmark initial 2015 trials and extended-window trials (DAWN, DEFUSE 3) for EVT selected patients based on the concept of adequate salvageable tissue, either by CT ASPECTS > 6, or on tissue-at-risk criteria by perfusion imaging. For DAWN, the ischemic core cutoffs were <21 mL (age > 80) and <31 mL (age < 80). DEFUSE 3 used initial ischemic core cutoff of <70 mL.[9-13,29,30]

Given the underrepresentation of patients with large initial strokes in the initial EVT trials and multiple posthoc analyses that were suggestive of the benefit of EVT in patients with large core infarcts, several RCTs were conducted to investigate.

The Recovery by Endovascular Salvage for Cerebral Ultra-acute Embolism Japan Large Ischemic Core Trial (RESCUE-Japan LIMIT) randomized 203 patients with CT or MR ASPECTS 3-5, with MRI being used for assessment in 86% of patients. 90-day mRS 0-2 was higher in the EVT group (14% vs. 7.8%), without significant differences in mortality or sICH between the two groups.[31]

The Endovascular Therapy in Acute Anterior Circulation Large Vessel Occlusion Patients with a Large Infract Core (ANGEL-ASPECT) trial randomized 456 patients with large core infarcts (including ASPECTS 0-2 and CTP core infarct volume of 70-100 mL). This study found that 90-day mRS 0-2 was superior in the EVT arm (30% vs. 11.6%). The rates of sICH were higher in the EVT group (6.1% vs. 2.7%), but the overall rate was comparable to most other EVT trials.[32]

The Randomized Controlled Trial to Optimize Patient's Selection for Endovascular Treatment in Acute Ischemic Stroke (SELECT2) enrolled 352 patients with anterior circulation large core strokes, defined as ASPECTS 3-5 or CTP core infarct volume > 50 mL. The primary outcome of 90-day mRS 0-2 was achieved in a significantly higher proportion of patients undergoing EVT (20% vs. 7%). There was no difference in the rates of sICH within the two groups, with a slight trend toward mortality benefit. Of note, EVT reduced the number of mRS 5 patients by >50%.[33]

Three additional trials (TESLA, TENSION, and LASTE) have had their respective preliminary data presented, showing similar results as the other trials mentioned. TESLA, which enrolled 300 patients, although positive, demonstrated a smaller overall treatment effect of EVT (9.9%) compared to that in RESCUE-Japan LIMIT (18.3%), ANGEL-ASPECT (13.7%), and SELECT2 (19.2%).[34]

These studies have prompted revision of societal guidelines to adopt EVT as standard of care for patients with anterior circulation LVO, aged 18-85 years, presenting within 24 hours of last known well/symptom onset with large infarct cores, defined as ASPECTS 3–5 or core infarct volume of 70–149 mL as class I, level A evidence. In addition, studies have shown that along with benefits to clinical outcomes, there are socioeconomic benefits of treatment of large core infarct patients. The major benefits are due to cost savings due to significant decreases in mRS 4 and 5 patients. The benefits of EVT in large core infarct patients with ASPECTS 0–2, age > 85, and >24 hours from last known well are not conclusive.[34]

Thrombectomy Beyond 24 Hours

As described, EVT has become standard of care for most patients with LVOs within 24 hours of symptoms onset or last known well time. There is a dearth of data demonstrating the benefit of EVT, however, after this 24 hours period. Data is limited largely to small case series and retrospective analysis.

A recent systemic review of 12 studies, and 894 patients demonstrated the rate of favorable functional outcome in these cases was 40%, with no significant differences in favorable outcomes, 90-day mortality, or sICH rate among patients who underwent EVT < 24 hours versus > 24 hours, suggesting that EVT may be beneficial at even prolonged time windows.[35]

Selection of these patients must be made on a case-by-case basis, in conjunction with advanced imaging and specific patient factors, and with careful extrapolation of EVT trial data available.

Endovascular Therapy Techniques

The initial EVT trials demonstrating efficacy and establishing the treatment as standard of care predominantly utilized the usage of SRs to achieve recanalization. Soon after, the development of A Direct Aspiration First Pass Technique (ADAPT), also known as contact aspiration (CA), created a dichotomy amongst interventionalists based on technique. Of course, several different techniques have been described throughout the literature, including combination usage of SRs and aspiration catheters.

As technology continues to rapidly advance, both SRs and aspiration catheters have become more sophisticated, allowing a range of device sizes and catheter bores to facilitate revascularization. With rapid advances in technology, the overall successful recanalization rates, as measured by the Modified Thrombolysis in Cerebral Infarction Score (mTICI), have been increasing in time, with continuously increasing rates of first-pass success, i.e., achieving successful recanalization with the first thrombectomy attempt. There has been a good amount of study performed on thrombectomy techniques, but no clear winner in terms of efficacy has been determined.

Three randomized clinical trials have been performed comparing these techniques. The Contact Aspiration versus Stent Retriever for Successful Revascularization (ASTER) trial, ASTER2, and the Aspiration Thrombectomy Versus Stent-Retriever Thrombectomy as First-Line Approach for Large Vessel Occlusion (COMPASS) trials were performed to address this question. Taken together, these trials demonstrated that SR and CA techniques were essentially equivalent. Of note, ASTER2 demonstrated that the combined use of CA and SR techniques may offer slight advance in first-pass successful recanalization when compared to SR alone (86.2% vs. 72.3%, $p = 0.04$).[36-38]

Small meta-analyses conducted have suggested a slight superiority of CA in achieving successful recanalization rates in both anterior and posterior circulation LVO strokes. Meta-analyses focusing and DMVO suggest that application of SR-based techniques (whether alone or in conjunction with CA) may yield higher recanalization rates. These studies have demonstrated a concurrent higher risk of intraprocedural subarachnoid hemorrhage.[39,40]

There remains relative equivalence in the effectiveness of either technique. Therefore, EVT is likely to be most successful when an operator approaches each patient on a case-by-case basis considering anatomical and clinical factors and utilizes a technique with which the operator has experience and familiarity.

Acute Stenting in Acute Ischemic Stroke

Acute stenting, both cervical and intracranial, is typically utilized as rescue options in the setting of failed thrombectomy attempts. The most common causative etiologies are recalcitrant clots, underlying atherosclerotic disease, and vessel dissection. Most data assessing these techniques is of retrospective nature with comparisons being made to historical controls.

Tandem lesions, defined as intracranial occlusion in conjunction with cervical ICA disease with >70% underlying stenosis, complicates approximately 15% of EVT cases for AIS. Tandem occlusions have been shown to be associated with worse outcomes. The predominant pathophysiological etiology is extracranial ICA atherosclerotic plaque rupture with subsequent distal embolization. Other etiologies include ICA dissection and presence of carotid webs.[41]

There are two approaches of treating tandem lesions. The first approach involves treatment of the extracranial lesion first, via angioplasty alone or placement of a stent, followed by treatment of the intracranial lesion. The second approach involves prioritizing the intracranial occlusion, followed by treatment of the extracranial lesion. Based on the current literature, there is no superior approach. One hypothesis favors treatment of the intracranial occlusion first, when possible, to maximize collateral circulation while attending to the more proximal lesion. In certain cases, the extracranial lesion must be addressed first to facilitate the passage of catheters and devices.

In terms of extracranial treatment methods, the choices are medical management, angioplasty alone, and stenting. Most evidence to guide decision making comes from the TITAN and STRATIS registries. The TITAN registry data suggests that patients with treated with acute antiplatelet medications and acute stenting have more favorable outcomes than patients treated with angioplasty alone or patients with no endovascular extracranial carotid intervention. There were no significant differences noted in the rates of sICH in patients who received IVT versus those who did not.[42] The STRATIS registry data demonstrated that patients with tandem occlusions who underwent acute stenting demonstrated higher rates of good outcomes (mRS 0-2) without any significant differences in mortality or sICH.[43] Although reassuring, it is important to note that these analyses were retrospective in nature with small sample sizes. Prospective studies would be required to better understand the implications of acute cervical stenting. There are also no real guidelines on the periprocedural antiplatelet management, and therefore, it is important for operators to have a nuanced understanding of various antiplatelet agents.

Intracranial stenting has been a topic of debate in the interventional community since the SAMMPRIS trial, which demonstrated superiority of medical management in the treatment of intracranial atherosclerotic disease-related stenosis when compared to stenting with the Wingspan stent system. SAMMPRIS demonstrated a 23.9% composite periprocedural complication rate.[44] A more recent trial, WEAVE, evaluated postmarket surveillance data in patients treated with Wingspan who met United States Food and

Drug Administration (US FDA)-approved criteria. On interim review of 152 patients, this study demonstrated much lower periprocedural complication rates 2.6%.[45]

Intracranial stenting as a rescue therapy for refractory occlusion, however, has been shown in small case series and retrospective analysis to be relatively safe and effective, with suggestion of improved patient outcomes compared to patients who do not achieve recanalization, albeit with the caveat of slightly increased sICH rates (9-10%) when compared to control groups. There is much heterogeneity, however, in techniques, devices, and perceived indications for pursuing rescue stenting currently.[46]

SYSTEMS OF CARE

Direct to Angiography

Currently, the triage process of AIS patients largely happens in the field, followed by the emergency department (ED). The ED is a crucial stop that allows stabilization of the patient, imaging to be obtained, IVT to be administered, and the patient to be monitored while preparations are being made for EVT (either by transfer to a thrombectomy-capable center or by in-house thrombectomy at comprehensive stroke centers).

Attempts have been made to decrease the time to IVT and EVT (e.g., via utilization of mobile stroke units), and applying strict workflows to improve patient outcomes. Once such concept is the direct-to-angiography (DTA) approach. This approach involves triage from the field, mobile stroke unit, or initial receiving hospital, directly to a neuroangiography suite, where the patient can undergo imaging directly, receive IVT, and undergo thrombectomy if indicated, essentially bypassing the ED altogether.

There is mixed data to suggest utility of this approach. So far, one RCT, has been completed evaluating direct transfer. ANGIOCAT, which randomized 138 patients to a DTA approach or conventional approach, demonstrated reduced door-to-groin puncture times (18 vs. 42, $p < 0.001$) and improved clinical outcomes [adjust common odds ratio (OR) 2.2, 95 confidence interval (CI) 1.2–4.1; $p = 0.009$] with the DTA approach.[47] Several meta-analyses also support corroborate these findings, along with findings that a DTA approach may also allow for significant cost savings.[48]

Although encouraging, there are some obvious limitations. The first challenge is outfitting the neurointerventional team to manage patients regardless of their clinical status—clinically unstable patients may be better served with the expertise of emergency physicians in terms of securing airways, achieving hemodynamic stability, and management of concurrent conditions prior to arriving to the neuroangiography suite. Another challenge is advanced imaging. Although cone-beam CT is widely available throughout neuroangiography suites, perfusion imaging is not. For patients with large-core infarctions or DMVOs, this may present challenges in selection of patients. As such, effective implementation will require a multidisciplinary, streamlined approach, and continued efforts to understand the implications of DTA approaches **(Fig. 3)**.

Telestroke

Despite increasing awareness and recognition of stroke and available therapies, there remains significant barriers in access to stroke care. A large proportion of the general population does not have immediate access to a stroke center, stroke specialists, and IVT/EVT. Studies have shown, for example, that stroke mortality is significantly higher for rural patients compared to patients in urban areas.

Given these concerns, there has been tremendous grown in the field of telemedicine, namely telestroke. Telestroke technology is the utilization of remote phone

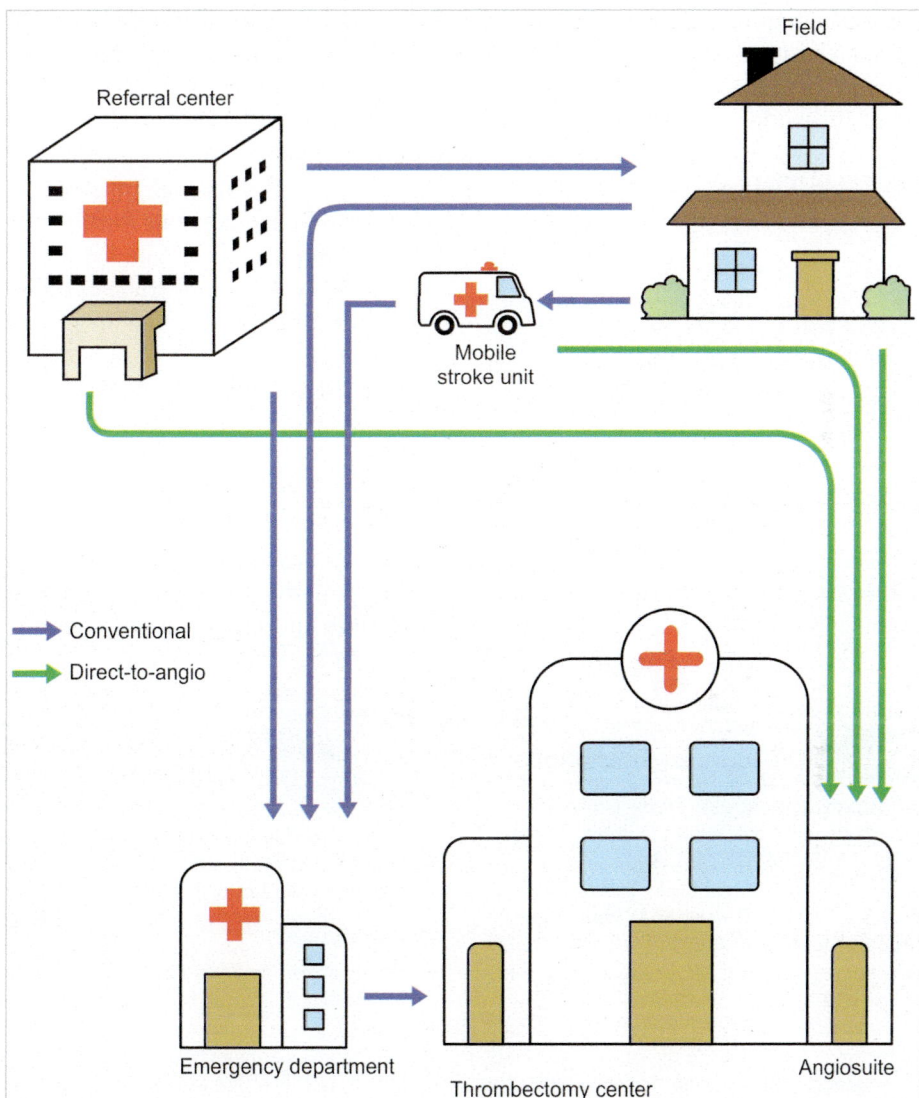

FIG. 3: Direct to angio transfer of LVO AIS as compared to conventional triage via emergency department.
(AIS: acute ischemic stroke; LVO: large vessel occlusion)

and video conferencing in delivering acute stroke care. A stroke physician can use this technology to virtually assess a patient and determine candidacy for IVT and EVT, and aid in arranging transfer to the appropriate level of care. This allows isolated facilities and regions to benefit from timely evaluation and treatment, principles that are paramount in AIS care.

Telestroke programs have been shown to improve mortality and health outcomes, increase IVT administration, reduce geographic and racial disparities in stroke treatment, and allow for cost benefits to the health system in general.[49,50] Although becoming more popular, these systems have yet to achieve widespread use, especially on the global stage. As such, more research is being conducted and efforts are being made to gain insight into effective integration of telestroke networks and infrastructure throughout the world.

CONCLUSION

In conclusion, the landscape of AIS care has evolved dramatically over the past few decades, largely driven by advancements in reperfusion and endovascular therapies. While the introduction of IVT in 1996 and EVT in 2015 marked significant milestones, ongoing research and clinical trials have continued to expand the eligible patient populations for these treatments. This evolution has been guided by a growing understanding of stroke pathophysiology, refinements in imaging techniques, and technological advancements in thrombectomy devices.

The expansion of treatment windows for IVT, exploration of its use in cases with low NIHSS, and the broadening of EVT applications to include patients with large cores, low NIHSS, posterior circulation LVO, and distal occlusions, all underscore the rapidly evolving indications for treatment of AIS. Accumulating evidence from ongoing clinical trials will inform which of these new approaches will lead to guideline changes in AIS treatment.

In addition to therapeutic interventions, innovations in stroke care systems, such as DTA and telestroke approaches, have emerged with the potential to streamline care delivery and improve patient outcomes. Their widespread implementation will depend on ongoing research to definitively prove their efficacy and optimize their effectiveness.

REFERENCES

1. National Institute of Neurological Disorders and Stroke rt-PA Stroke Study Group. Tissue plasminogen activator for acute ischemic stroke. N Engl J Med. 1995;333(24):1581-7.
2. Hacke W, Kaste M, Bluhmki E, Brozman M, Dávalos A, Guidetti D, et al; ECASS Investigators. Thrombolysis with alteplase 3 to 4.5 hours after acute ischemic stroke. N Engl J Med. 2008;359(13):1317-29.
3. Thomalla G, Simonsen CZ, Boutitie F, Andersen G, Berthezene Y, Cheng B, et al; WAKE-UP Investigators. MRI-Guided Thrombolysis for Stroke with Unknown Time of Onset. N Engl J Med. 2018;379(7):611-22.
4. Ma H, Campbell BCV, Parsons MW, Churilov L, Levi CR, Hsu C, et al; EXTEND Investigators. Thrombolysis Guided by Perfusion Imaging up to 9 Hours after Onset of Stroke. N Engl J Med. 2019;380(19):1795-803.
5. Albers GW, Jumaa M, Purdon B, Zaidi SF, Streib C, Shuaib A, et al; TIMELESS Investigators. Tenecteplase for Stroke at 4.5 to 24 Hours with Perfusion-Imaging Selection. N Engl J Med. 2024;390(8):701-11.
6. Xiong Y, Campbell BCV, Fisher M, Schwamm LH, Parsons M, Li H, et al. Rationale and design of Tenecteplase Reperfusion Therapy in Acute Ischaemic Cerebrovascular Events III (TRACE III): a randomised, phase III, open-label, controlled trial. Stroke Vasc Neurol. 2024;9(1):82-9.
7. Khatri P, Kleindorfer DO, Devlin T, Sawyer RN Jr, Starr M, Mejilla J, et al; PRISMS Investigators. Effect of Alteplase vs Aspirin on Functional Outcome for Patients With Acute Ischemic Stroke and Minor Nondisabling Neurologic Deficits: The PRISMS Randomized Clinical Trial. JAMA. 2018;320(2):156-66.
8. Romano JG, Gardener H, Campo-Bustillo I, Khan Y, Riley N, Tai S, et al. The Mild and Rapidly Improving Stroke Study (MaRISS): Rationale and design. Int J Stroke. 2019;14(9):983-6.
9. Fransen PS, Beumer D, Berkhemer OA, van den Berg LA, Lingsma H, van der Lugt A, et al; MR CLEAN Investigators. MR CLEAN, a multicenter randomized clinical trial of endovascular treatment for acute ischemic stroke in the Netherlands: study protocol for a randomized controlled trial. Trials. 2014;15:343.
10. Saver JL, Goyal M, Bonafe A, Diener HC, Levy EI, Pereira VM, et al; SWIFT PRIME Investigators. Solitaire™ with the Intention for Thrombectomy as Primary Endovascular Treatment for Acute Ischemic Stroke (SWIFT PRIME) trial: protocol for a randomized, controlled, multicenter study

comparing the Solitaire revascularization device with IV tPA with IV tPA alone in acute ischemic stroke. Int J Stroke. 2015;10(3):439-48.
11. Molina CA, Chamorro A, Rovira À, de Miquel A, Serena J, Roman LS, et al. REVASCAT: a randomized trial of revascularization with SOLITAIRE FR device vs. best medical therapy in the treatment of acute stroke due to anterior circulation large vessel occlusion presenting within eight-hours of symptom onset. Int J Stroke. 2015;10(4):619-26.
12. Campbell BC, Mitchell PJ, Kleinig TJ, Dewey HM, Churilov L, Yassi N, et al; EXTEND-IA Investigators. Endovascular therapy for ischemic stroke with perfusion-imaging selection. N Engl J Med. 2015;372(11):1009-18.
13. Goyal M, Demchuk AM, Menon BK, Eesa M, Rempel JL, Thornton J, et al; ESCAPE Trial Investigators. Randomized assessment of rapid endovascular treatment of ischemic stroke. N Engl J Med. 2015;372(11):1019-30.
14. Raha O, Hall C, Malik A, D'Anna L, Lobotesis K, Kwan J, et al. Advances in mechanical thrombectomy for acute ischaemic stroke. BMJ Med. 2023;2(1):e000407.
15. Siegler JE, Albright KC, George AJ, Boehme AK, Gillette MA, Kumar AD, et al. Time to Neurological Deterioration in Ischemic Stroke. Med Student Res J. 2017;4:18-24.
16. Lin CH, Saver JL, Ovbiagele B, Tang SC, Lee M, Liebeskind DS. Effects of endovascular therapy for mild stroke due to proximal or M2 occlusions: meta-analysis. J Neurointerv Surg. 2023;15(4):350-4.
17. Kobeissi H, Bilgin C, Ghozy S, Kadirvel R, Kallmes DF, Brinjikji W. A review of acute ischemic stroke caused by distal, medium vessel occlusions. Interv Neuroradiol. 2023:15910199231197616.
18. Saver JL, Chapot R, Agid R, Hassan A, Jadhav AP, Liebeskind DS, et al; Distal Thrombectomy Summit Group*†. Thrombectomy for Distal, Medium Vessel Occlusions: A Consensus Statement on Present Knowledge and Promising Directions. Stroke. 2020;51(9):2872-84.
19. Lau HL, Gardener H, Coutts SB, Saini V, Field TS, Dowlatshahi D, et al. Radiographic characteristics of mild ischemic stroke patients with visible intracranial occlusion: The INTERRSeCT Study. Stroke. 2022;53(3):913-20.
20. Alaka SA, Menon BK, Brobbey A, Williamson T, Goyal M, Demchuk AM, et al. Functional Outcome Prediction in Ischemic Stroke: A Comparison of Machine Learning Algorithms and Regression Models. Front Neurol. 2020;11:889.
21. Nogueira RG, Doheim MF, Al-Bayati AR, Lee JS, Haussen DC, Mohammaden M, et al. Distal medium vessel occlusion strokes: Understanding the present and paving the way for a better future. J Stroke. 2024;26(2):190-202.
22. Ospel JM, Goyal M. A review of endovascular treatment for medium vessel occlusion stroke. J Neurointerv Surg. 2021;13:623-30.
23. Anadani M, Alawieh A, Chalhoub R, Jabbour P, Starke RM, Arthur A, et al. Mechanical thrombectomy for distal occlusions: efficacy, functional and safety outcomes: insight from the STAR collaboration. World Neurosurg. 2021;151:e871-9.
24. Baik SH, Kim JY, Jung C. A review of endovascular treatment for posterior circulation strokes. Neurointervention. 2023;18(2):90-106.
25. Liu X, Dai Q, Ye R, Zi W, Liu Y, Wang H, et al; BEST Trial Investigators. Endovascular treatment versus standard medical treatment for vertebrobasilar artery occlusion (BEST): An open-label, randomised controlled trial. Lancet Neurol. 2020;19(2):115-22.
26. Schonewille WJ, Wijman CA, Michel P, Rueckert CM, Weimar C, Mattle HP, et al; BASICS Study Group. Treatment and outcomes of acute basilar artery occlusion in the Basilar Artery International Cooperation Study (BASICS): A prospective registry study. Lancet Neurol. 2009;8:724-30.
27. Jovin TG, Li C, Wu L, Wu C, Chen J, Jiang C, et al; BAOCHE Investigators. Trial of Thrombectomy 6 to 24 Hours after Stroke Due to Basilar-Artery Occlusion. N Engl J Med. 2022;387(15):1373-84.
28. Tao C, Li R, Zhu Y, Qun S, Xu P, Wang L, et al. Endovascular treatment for acute basilar artery occlusion: A multicenter randomized controlled trial (ATTENTION). Int J Stroke. 2022;17(7):815-9.
29. Nogueira RG, Jadhav AP, Haussen DC, Bonafe A, Budzik RF, Bhuva P, et al; DAWN Trial Investigators. Thrombectomy 6 to 24 Hours after Stroke with a Mismatch between Deficit and Infarct. N Engl J Med. 2018;378(1):11-21.
30. Albers GW, Marks MP, Kemp S, Christensen S, Tsai JP, Ortega-Gutierrez S, et al; DEFUSE 3 Investigators. Thrombectomy for Stroke at 6 to 16 Hours with Selection by Perfusion Imaging. N Engl J Med. 2018;378(8):708-18.
31. Yoshimura S, Uchida K, Sakai N, Yamagami H, Inoue M, Toyoda K, et al. Randomized Clinical Trial of Endovascular Therapy for Acute Large Vessel Occlusion with Large Ischemic Core (RESCUE-Japan LIMIT): Rationale and Study Protocol. Neurol Med Chir (Tokyo). 2022;62(3):156-64.
32. Huo X, Ma G, Tong X, Zhang X, Pan Y, Nguyen TN,; ANGEL-ASPECT Investigators. Trial of Endovascular

Therapy for Acute Ischemic Stroke with Large Infarct. N Engl J Med. 2023;388(14):1272-83.
33. Sarraj A, Hassan AE, Abraham MG, Ortega-Gutierrez S, Kasner SE, Hussain MS, et al; SELECT2 Investigators. Trial of Endovascular Thrombectomy for Large Ischemic Strokes. N Engl J Med. 2023;388(14):1259-71.
34. Al-Mufti F, Marden FA, Burkhardt JK, Raper D, Schirmer CM, Baker A, et al; SNIS Standards and Guidelines Committee; SNIS Board of Directors. Endovascular therapy for anterior circulation emergent large vessel occlusion stroke in patients with large ischemic cores: A report of the SNIS Standards and Guidelines Committee. J Neurointerv Surg. 2024:jnis-2023-021444.
35. Rodriguez-Calienes A, Galecio-Castillo M, Vivanco-Suarez J, Mohamed GA, Toth G, Sarraj A, et al. Endovascular thrombectomy beyond 24 hours from last known well: A systematic review with meta-analysis. J Neurointerv Surg. 2024;16(7):670-6.
36. Lapergue B, Blanc R, Gory B, Labreuche J, Duhamel A, Marnat G, et al; ASTER Trial Investigators. Effect of Endovascular Contact Aspiration vs Stent Retriever on Revascularization in Patients With Acute Ischemic Stroke and Large Vessel Occlusion: The ASTER Randomized Clinical Trial. JAMA. 2017;318(5):443-52.
37. Lapergue B, Blanc R, Costalat V, Desal H, Saleme S, Spelle L, et al; ASTER2 Trial Investigators. Effect of Thrombectomy With Combined Contact Aspiration and Stent Retriever vs Stent Retriever Alone on Revascularization in Patients With Acute Ischemic Stroke and Large Vessel Occlusion: The ASTER2 Randomized Clinical Trial. JAMA. 2021;326(12):1158-69.
38. Turk AS 3rd, Siddiqui A, Fifi JT, De Leacy RA, Fiorella DJ, Gu E, et al. Aspiration thrombectomy versus stent retriever thrombectomy as first-line approach for large vessel occlusion (COMPASS): A multicentre, randomised, open label, blinded outcome, non-inferiority trial. Lancet. 2019;393(10175):998-1008.
39. Kaneko N, Sakuta K, Imahori T, Gedion H, Ghovvati M, Tateshima S. Devices and Techniques. J Neuroendovasc Ther. 2023;17(11):257-62.
40. Munoz A, Jabre R, Orenday-Barraza JM, Eldin MS, Chen CJ, Al-Saiegh F, et al. A review of mechanical thrombectomy techniques for acute ischemic stroke. Interv Neuroradiol. 2023;29(4):450-8.
41. Di Donna A, Muto G, Giordano F, Muto M, Guarnieri G, Servillo G, et al. Diagnosis and management of tandem occlusion in acute ischemic stroke. Eur J Radiol Open. 2023;11:100513.
42. Anadani M, Spiotta AM, Alawieh A, Turjman F, Piotin M, Haussen DC, et al; TITAN (Thrombectomy In TANdem Lesions) Investigators. Emergent Carotid Stenting Plus Thrombectomy After Thrombolysis in Tandem Strokes: Analysis of the TITAN Registry. Stroke. 2019;50(8):2250-2.
43. Jadhav AP, Zaidat OO, Liebeskind DS, Yavagal DR, Haussen DC, Hellinger FR Jr, et al. Emergent Management of Tandem Lesions in Acute Ischemic Stroke. Stroke. 2019;50(2):428-33.
44. Chimowitz MI, Lynn MJ, Derdeyn CP, Turan TN, Fiorella D, Lane BF, et al; SAMMPRIS Trial Investigators. Stenting versus aggressive medical therapy for intracranial arterial stenosis. N Engl J Med. 2011;365(11):993-1003.
45. Alexander MJ, Zauner A, Gupta R, Alshekhlee A, Fraser JF, Toth G, et al. The WOVEN trial: Wingspan One-year Vascular Events and Neurologic Outcomes. J Neurointerv Surg. 2021;13(4):307-10.
46. Alexander MJ, Yu W. Intracranial atherosclerosis update for neurointerventionalists. J Neurointerv Surg. 2024;16(5):522-8.
47. Requena M, Olivé-Gadea M, Muchada M, Hernández D, Rubiera M, Boned S, et al. Direct to Angiography Suite Without Stopping for Computed Tomography Imaging for Patients With Acute Stroke: A Randomized Clinical Trial. JAMA Neurol. 2021;78(9):1099-107.
48. Desai SM, Psychogios M, Khatri P, Jovin TG, Jadhav AP. Direct Transfer to the Neuroangiography Suite for Patients With Stroke. Stroke. 2023;54(6):1674-84.
49. Jauch EC, Schwamm LH, Panagos PD, Barbazzeni J, Dickson R, Dunne R, et al; Prehospital Stroke System of Care Consensus Conference. Recommendations for Regional Stroke Destination Plans in Rural, Suburban, and Urban Communities From the Prehospital Stroke System of Care Consensus Conference: A Consensus Statement From the American Academy of Neurology, American Heart Association/American Stroke Association, American Society of Neuroradiology, National Association of EMS Physicians, National Association of State EMS Officials, Society of NeuroInterventional Surgery, and Society of Vascular and Interventional Neurology: Endorsed by the Neurocritical Care Society. Stroke. 2021;52(5):e133-52.
50. Demaerschalk BM, Berg J, Chong BW, Gross H, Nystrom K, Adeoye O, et al. American Telemedicine Association: Telestroke Guidelines. Telemed J E Health. 2017;23(5):376-89.

CHAPTER 6

Management of Direct-acting Oral Anticoagulant–Associated Intracerebral Hemorrhage

Sucharita Ray, Kamalesh Chakravarty

ABSTRACT

Direct-acting oral anticoagulants (DOACs) find increasing usage for their advantage over traditional anticoagulants. Reliable action and pharmacokinetic profile and obviating the need for monitoring are the major advantages. However, bleeding, especially intracerebral hemorrhage remains a small but significant complication. Reported numbers are likely to increase as the overall usage of DOACs increases and this makes it imperative to fill the extant knowledge gaps in their management. This chapter discusses the existing evidence around the management of intracerebral hemorrhage due to DOACs.

Keywords: DOACs, Pharmacokinetic, Management, Evidence, Intracerebral hemorrhage.

INTRODUCTION

Newer direct-acting oral anticoagulants (DOACs) are now the preferred drug for secondary stroke prophylaxis in nonvalvular atrial fibrillation and in patients with venous thromboembolism. Their use is justified through their predictable pharmacokinetics as well as improved safety profile over coumarin anticoagulants **(Fig. 1)**. DOACs are variably bound to proteins and this determines their activity and elimination. Reduced renal function also requires drug modification as many DOACs are excreted renally.[1] The other advantage that DOACs over coumarin anticoagulants are that they do not require frequent monitoring of international normalized ratio (INR) for adjudging efficacy and ruling out toxicity **(Fig. 1)**.

Despite these advantages, hemorrhage remains the single most important side effect of DOACs. DOACs have been associated with an overall lesser rate of bleeding as compared to warfarin and similar agents. The rate of all bleeding [including major hemorrhage, fatal hemorrhage, hemorrhagic stroke, or intracerebral hemorrhage (ICH)] is lower for DOACs at 3–4% as compared to warfarin with rates of 5–6%. ICH rates for DOACs have been calculated to be 0.3–0.4% versus 0.7–0.8% for warfarin. Due to increased usage of DOACs over time, data from a nationally representative public health surveillance system showed the period 2016–2020 showed an increase in DOAC-related bleeding incidents compared to warfarin (27.9% vs. 8.8%).[2] For this reason, there is a need to monitor the pharmacokinetic and pharmacodynamic effects in the body as well as find agents to suitably neutralize the effects in cases of overdose or unacceptable side effects in the users.

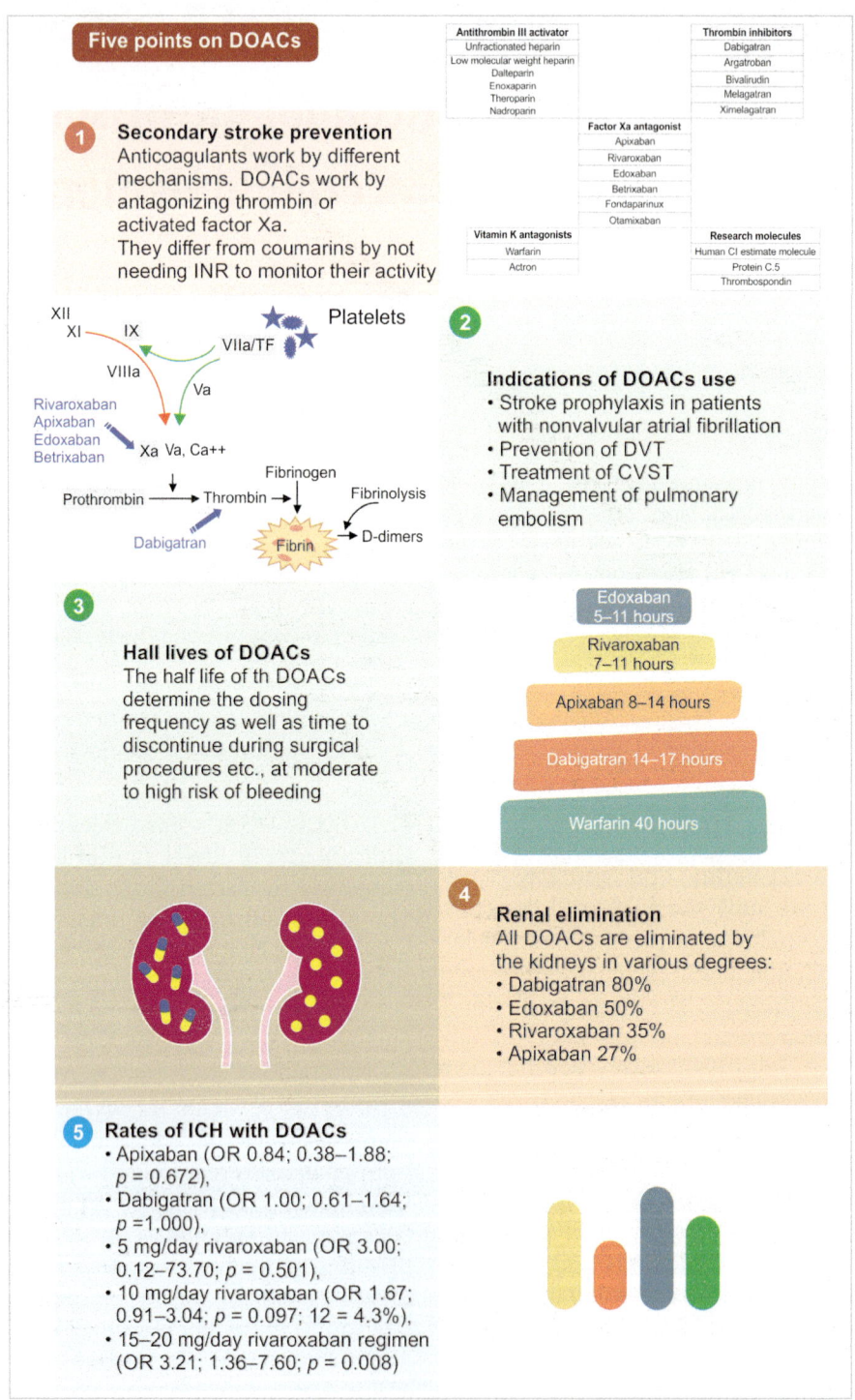

FIG. 1: Infographic on DOACs use in clinical practice.
(CVST: cerebral venous sinus thrombosis; DOACs: direct acting anticoagulants; DVT: deep venous thrombosis)

This chapter will have a brief discussion on the mechanism of action of DOACs, and evidence-based management of NOAC-associated bleeding with special reference to intracranial hemorrhage.

■ MECHANISM OF ACTION

The DOACs act by the direct inhibition of factors in the clotting cascade. Dabigatran was one of the earliest agents to be introduced as a DOAC which acted by inhibition of thrombin. Later other molecules targeting factor Xa were developed. Today, a variety of molecules acting by antagonizing factor Xa and thrombin are used for secondary stroke prophylaxis. Amongst the thrombin inhibitors, dabigatran was one of the first molecules to be developed that act as a competitive antagonist of factor II.[3] On the other hand, argatroban, a synthetic competitive thrombin inhibitor used parenterally.[4] Similarly, factor Xa antagonists have been approved for use for secondary stroke prophylaxis in patients with nonvalvular atrial fibrillation and prevention against systemic embolism as well for prophylaxis against cerebral and deep vein thrombosis. These agents have become popular compared to the vitamin K antagonists (VKAs) due to requiring less monitoring, favorable side effect profile, and less risk of hemorrhage.

■ INTRACEREBRAL HEMORRHAGE DUE TO DIRECT-ACTING ORAL ANTICOAGULANTS

Even though DOACs reduce the risk of hemorrhage by about 56% compared to VKAs intracranial hemorrhage remains one of the most serious complications associated with DOACs.[5] There is very little data on how the hematoma due to a DOAC differs from that caused due to a VKA. Bleeding risk has been found to vary for different agents. A cross-sectional observational study of all ICH caused by patients on oral anticoagulants found that when compared to warfarin the ICH caused by DOACs was less likely to impair consciousness (31.3% vs. 39.4%; $p = 0.002$) or require surgical clearance (5.3% vs. 9.9%;[5] $p = 0.024$). Overall mortality too was significantly less with NOACs as compared to warfarin.[6] A meta-analysis of randomized trials comparing the NOACs for the risk of ICH found similar bleeding risk for apixaban, dabigatran, and 5 and 10 mg doses of rivaroxaban when compared to aspirin. However, rates of ICH were higher in the 20 mg rivaroxaban group.[7] Intracranial bleeding is often the most common cause of bleeding due to inappropriate high doses of these agents.[8] Some recent research has focused on the friability of the clot due to DOACs and how it differs from those caused by VKAs.

Although the popularity of DOAC rests on not requiring the monitoring of drug levels or coagulation parameters, the pharmacokinetic differences between individuals and within individuals are not known. Variations in drug levels may explain a difference in the individual levels. Hence some have advocated estimation of drug levels by antifactor Xa concentrations and diluted thrombin time (TT) (dabigatran) to be a good measure of the drug levels in individuals.[9]

■ CHARACTERISTICS OF DIRECT-ACTING ORAL ANTICOAGULANT-INDUCED INTRACEREBRAL HEMORRHAGE

Anticoagulant-associated hemorrhages have a special predilection to the cerebellum. Previous acute ischemic strokes, coronary artery disease, atrial fibrillation, and deep vein thrombosis were other predictors of the condition.[10]

Overall incidence of DOAC-associated ICH has been reported to vary with different agents. In comparison to low-molecular-weight heparins (LMWHs), most DOACs (apixaban, edoxaban, and rivaroxaban) had a similar risk of ICH. However, in comparison with aspirin, dabigatran and apixaban had a similar risk of ICH, while rivaroxaban posed an increased risk of ICH [risk ratio (RR) 2.12; 95% confidence interval (CI) 1.31–3.44].[11]

A nationwide Japanese survey exploring characteristics of ICH due to DOAC versus vitamin K anticoagulant shows that DOAC-associated ICH was less likely to cause impaired consciousness (31.3% vs. 39.4%, $p = 0.002$) or require surgical evacuation (5.3% vs. 9.9%, $p = 0.024$). Patients with warfarin-induced ICH are also more likely to face increased rates of 1 and 7-day mortality as compared to those on DOAC.[6]

General Measures of Management

There is a need for knowledge of proper prescription and dosing of DOACs in indicated patients. Although DOACs have been associated with less incidence of overt bleeding as compared to traditional anticoagulants, hospital trends show a higher number of emergency visits by patients in recent years. Increased survival may be the biggest cofounder in this study, but there is a need to have proper knowledge of the choice of DOAC and appropriate dose to be used for anticoagulation.[2]

General measures for the management of patients with DOAC-induced ICH hinge on supportive measures such as stabilization of the patient, maintenance of airway and breathing, and monitoring of vitals. Any overt bleeding elsewhere in the body must be noted as they may accompany ICH. Proper venous access and telemetry should be instituted and signs of raised intracranial pressure, impending herniation, etc. should be noted. Concurrent antiplatelets, antihypertensives, and other medications should be noted.

Background Information

Acute management of DOAC-induced ICH requires a proper assessment of the severity of the bleeding. It is crucial to know the volume of the bleed, and the neurological status of the patient, a proper clinical examination to assess the stroke severity on National Institutes of Health Stroke Scale (NIHSS) as well as the anticipated final volume of the bleeding. A number of studies have proven that DOAC-induced ICH is neither associated with increased mortality nor expansion of bleeds as compared to VKAs.[12] It is vital to note the type and the last dose of DOAC at the time of presentation. Rivaroxaban displays high bioavailability when consumed with food as compared to when taken on an empty stomach.[13] Renal elimination is also a major determinant of drug action **(Fig. 1)**. Additionally, a mean of a minimum of four half-lives needs to have crossed before drug action may be considered to have ceased.[14]

Assessment of Direct-acting Oral Anticoagulant Action

Evaluation of dilute TT or ecarin clotting time are validated tests for assessment of thrombin inhibitors. Prolongation of activated partial thromboplastin time (aPTT) indicated the presence of dabigatran, but it is not as sensitive as TT.[15] Chromogenic antifactor IIa assay is also used to assess thrombin action. Assessment of antifactor Xa activity is used for apixaban and rivaroxaban. Additionally, serum drug levels can also be used for the assessment of individual drugs.[16] Many of the centers do not have the facilities for measurement of DOACs at this stage. A drug concentration > 50 ng/mL is sufficient to warrant reversal in patients with serious bleeding, and this limit may be relaxed to 30 ng/mL in those who require urgent intervention.[17] The culprit DOAC should also be discontinued until further reversal and resolution of the bleeding.

MANAGEMENT OF BLOOD PRESSURE

Blood pressure lowering is a potential target to prevent the growth of hematoma. Guidelines to reduce blood pressure have evolved in the last two decades. Earlier the guidelines recommended a blood pressure lowering to the level of 180 mm Hg systolic.[15] Later, results of the ATACH-2 trial and INTERACT-2 trial showed that lowering systolic blood pressure to <140 mm Hg within 1 hour showed lowered modified Rankin scores for the intensive group versus guideline recommended lowering.[15] There are no definite head-to-head trials about blood pressure targets in patients on anticoagulants, and the ATACH-2 trial excluded patients on DOACs. However, adequate reduction of blood pressure should be ensured in these groups of patients with close evaluation of vitals and clinical status.

REVERSAL OF DIRECT-ACTING ORAL ANTICOAGULANT ACTION

Reversal of DOAC action depends on the use of specific agents as well as nonspecific reversal. The reversal agents have evolved over the years. **Table 1** gives a comparative table for the difference between the common reversal agents used to reverse DOAC action.
- *Fresh frozen plasma (FFP)*: FFP and prothrombin complex concentrate

TABLE 1: Reversal agents for direct acting oral anticoagulants.

	Nonspecific agents		Specific reversal and bypassing agents		
	Prothrombin complex concentrate	Recombinant factor VIIa	Idarucizumab	Andexanet alfa	Ciraparantag
Agent	Concentrate of II, VII, IX, and X	Factor VIIa	Humanized monoclonal antibody fragment against dabigatran	Recombinant human factor Xa variant	Synthetic small molecule that has procoagulant activity not suppressible by Xa antagonists
Dosing	25–50 IU/kg or fixed dose of 2,000 IU intravenously 50–100 IU/kg intravenously if activated complex concentrate	15–90 µg/kg intravenously	5 g bolus intravenously	• *Low dose:* 400 mg IV over 15 minutes followed by an infusion of 480 mg over 2 hours (4 mg/min) • *High dose:* 800 mg IV over 15 minutes followed by an infusion of 960 mg over 2 hours (8 mg/min)	Intravenously (optimal dose unknown)
Half-life	Ranges from 4–6 hours (factor VII) to 60 hours (factor II)	2–3 hours	• Initial: ~45 minutes • Terminal: 4–8 hours	~4 hours	12–19 minutes
Prothrombotic effects	Yes	Yes	No	Yes (inhibition of tissue factor pathway inhibitor)	Unknown

(PCC) are the nonspecific agents used to control bleeding. FFP was the first agent to be used primarily for warfarin reversal before the advent of PCC. It usually has a large volume per session and has to undergo thawing before administration. The reversal of anticoagulant action takes more time. It has no role in the reversal of DOACs.[15]

- *PCC*: It is one of the most common hemostatic agents used to reverse the anticoagulant action. One of the main reasons for its popularity is that specific agents are costly and not widely available. It is available in two forms, three-factor PCC (3-PCC) containing factors II, IX, and X, or four-factor PCC (4-PCC) containing factors II, VII, IX, and X. PCC is primarily used to reverse warfarin-induced intracranial bleeding by supplementing the vitamin K containing factors in the blood. Its hemostatic efficacy in reversing anticoagulant action in DOAC-associated ICH is not known. A small retrospective study studying a fixed lower dose of 4-PCC (25 U/kg) against the recommended 50 U/kg showed high levels of hemostatic efficacy in reversing anticoagulant action. However, two patients developed thromboembolic complications. However, it is unclear if this hemostatic efficacy is associated with improved functional outcomes. A separate retrospective cohort study in Chinese patients showed efficacy of 4-PCC in a dose of 25–50 IU/kg versus conservative management. The study failed to associate 4-PCC with improved neurological recovery, 90-day mortality, in-hospital mortality, or reduced hematoma expansion. The 4-PCC has a higher concentration of clotting factors and was associated with a higher incidence of thromboembolic events in comparison to FFP in a comparative chart review (17.7% versus 2.7%).[18]
- *Factor VIIa*: It has not been seen to be effective in correcting aPTT or TT in dabigatran of antifactor Xa levels in rivaroxaban, but correction of prolonged PT in rivaroxaban has been reported. The use of activated factor VII is not recommended in the reversal of DOACs.[15]
- *Hemodialysis*: It reduces the serum concentration of dabigatran in refractory cases of bleeding. However, the process is cumbersome and difficult to access and must be utilized in refractory bleeding secondary to dabigatran overuse or patients with renal injury. Activated charcoal may sometimes be used to prevent intestinal absorption of dabigatran.[19]
- *Idarucizumab*: Among the specific molecules, monoclonal antibodies have been developed against dabigatran and other factor Xa antagonists. Idarucizumab is a humanized monoclonal antibody to neutralizes the action of dabigatran, a direct thrombin inhibitor. A prospective cohort study of 90 patients showed reversal of dabigatran-induced anticoagulation in 88–98% of the patients, the reversal taking only a few minutes to be effective. The activity of dabigatran was measured by elevations in the dilute TT and ecarin clotting time.[20] This trial was followed by the landslide REVERSE-AD trial which showed safe, near 100% reversal of dabigatran reversal with idarucizumab. A recent meta-analysis evaluating the efficacy of reversal with idarucizumab showed hemostatic efficacy in 77.7% and normal periprocedural hemostasis in 98.5%. The pooled incidences of all-cause mortality were 13.6% and that for thromboembolic events at any follow-up duration was 2.0% (95% CI 0.8–3.4%), respectively.[21]
- *Andexanet alfa*: It is a recombinant, inactive form of factor Xa that binds all inhibitors of factor Xa including heparins.

Two preliminary trials ANNEXA-A and ANNEXA-R utilizing the use of andexanet alfa in volunteers on apixaban and rivaroxaban showed near 90% reduction in levels after a single bolus dose, with a wearing off time of 2 hours. These trials paved the way for approval of andexanet alfa for use in these two drugs.[22] The agent was subsequently given approval by the FDA in 2018. The ANNEXA-I trial is a randomized control trial that compared the hemostatic efficacy of patients on andexanet alfa compared to conservative management, 85.5% of which received 4-PCC. Hemostatic efficacy difference with andexanet was 67% versus 53.1% with a mean difference in levels of decrease in antifactor Xa at 1–2 hours was 94.5%. Patients in the intervention arm showed thrombotic events in 10.3% of patients versus 5.6% in the control arm.[23] In this study, thrombotic events were seen to the extent of 10.2% which was also similar to the single arm andexanet study. This shows a possible prothrombotic effect of andexanet through the binding of tissue factor pathway inhibitor, which also increases levels of D-dimer and prothrombin levels.[23]

Andexanet alfa is now prescribed for various indications—prevention of deep venous thrombosis, secondary stroke prophylaxis in nonvalvular atrial fibrillation, treatment of deep venous thrombosis, etc. The dose of andexanet alfa needs to be modified according to the timing and size of the last dose **(Table 2)**.

- *Ciraparantag*: It is effective against all factor Xa antagonists as well as heparins. It is a synthetic molecule that shows noncovalent binding to direct Xa inhibitors, direct thrombin inhibitors, and unfractionated and LMWHs. The original molecule and its metabolites are almost completely excreted in the urine. However, it does not bind to coagulation factors and commonly used drugs. It is being developed as a universal anticoagulant reversal agent due to these properties.[24]
- *Factor XIa inhibitors*: These are the latest molecules on the dock that prevent the action of activated factor XIa in the indirect pathway. These drugs have been considered to be both antithrombotic, as well as anticoagulant in their mode of action given their site of action. Asundexian and milvexian are small molecule inhibitors of factor XIa whereas fesomersen, abelacimab, osocimab, and xisomab are monoclonal antibodies against factor XIa. PACIFIC-

TABLE 2: Dosing regimens for andexanet alfa for reversal of anticoagulant action.

Summary of andexanet alfa dosing reversal based on timing and size of last dose			
Factor Xa inhibitor	Last dose	Timing of last dose before andexanet alfa infusion < 8 hours or unknown	> 8 hours
Apixaban	<5 mg	Low dose	Low dose
	>5 mg/unknow	High dose	
Rivaroxaban	≤10 mg	Low dose	Low dose
	>10 mg/unknown	High dose	

Andexanet alfa infusion dose: *(Please also see Table 1)*
- *Low dose*: 400 mg (rate 30 mg/min) bolus and 4 mg/min for 120 minutes infusion
- *High dose*: 800 mg (rate 30 mg/min) bolus and 8 mg/min for 120 minutes infusion

STROKE was a randomized, placebo control, phase IIb trial that compared asundexian to a placebo for the prevention of atherothrombotic stroke. FXIa inhibition with asundexian did not reduce the composite of covert brain infarction or ischemic stroke. However, it also did not increase the composite of major or clinically relevant nonmajor bleeding compared with placebo in patients with acute, noncardioembolic ischemic stroke.[25] Similar results were also obtained for the AXIOMATIC-SSP trial using milvexian.[26] Future studies are required to study their role in stroke prevention and reversal agents based on factor XIa inhibition.

Resumption of Direct-acting Oral Anticoagulant Action after Reversal

The decision for patients to resume anticoagulation after DOAC reversal hinges on the risk factor profile, hematoma characterization, and rebound thrombotic complications of the reversal agents. There is no large-scale data regarding the same. In patients who developed ICH and had nonvalvular atrial fibrillation, early resumption of DOAC was no more harmful than later use for the development of ICH. 50% of the patients were on antiplatelet in this trial but this trial excluded patients on therapeutic anticoagulation. As of now, we need more comparative data of patients on therapeutic DOACs requiring reversal agents for ICH.

CONCLUSION

There is increased use of DOACs in reversing anticoagulant action. Judicious use of these agents needs to be explored to devise better management protocols and ensure better results in managing the devastating complications of these lifesaving drugs.

REFERENCES

1. Le Roux P, Pollack CV, Milan M, Schaefer A. Race against the clock: overcoming challenges in the management of anticoagulant-associated intracerebral hemorrhage. J Neurosurg. 2014;121 Suppl:1-20.
2. Geller AI, Shehab N, Lovegrove MC, Weidle NJ, Budnitz DS. Bleeding related to oral anticoagulants: Trends in US emergency department visits, 2016–2020. Thromb Res. 2023; 225:110-5.
3. Ganetsky M, Babu KM, Salhanick SD, Brown RS, Boyer EW. Dabigatran: Review of pharmacology and management of bleeding complications of this novel oral anticoagulant. J Med Toxicol. 2011;7(4):281-7.
4. McKeage K, Plosker GL. Argatroban. Drugs. 2001;61(4):515-22; discussion 523-524.
5. Caldeira D, Barra M, Pinto FJ, Ferreira JJ, Costa J. Intracranial hemorrhage risk with the new oral anticoagulants: a systematic review and meta-analysis. J Neurol. 2015;262(3):516-22.
6. Kurogi R, Nishimura K, Nakai M, Kada A, Kamitani S, Nakagawara J, et al. Comparing intracerebral hemorrhages associated with direct oral anticoagulants or warfarin. Neurology. 2018;90(13):e1143-9.
7. Mavrakanas TA, Charytan DM, Winkelmayer WC. Direct oral anticoagulants in CKD: An update. Curr Opin Nephrol Hypertens. 2020;29(5):489-96.
8. Jakowenko N, Nguyen S, Ruegger M, Dinh A, Salazar E, Donahue KR. Apixaban and rivaroxaban anti-Xa level utilization and associated bleeding events within an academic health system. Thromb Res. 2020;196:276-82.
9. Toorop MMA, van Rein N, Nierman MC, Vermaas HW, Huisman MV, van der Meer FJM, et al. Inter- and intra-individual concentrations of direct oral anticoagulants: The KIDOAC study. J Thromb Haemost. 2022;20(1):92-103.
10. Flaherty ML, Kissela B, Woo D, Kleindorfer D, Alwell K, Sekar P, et al. The increasing incidence of anticoagulant-associated intracerebral hemorrhage. Neurology. 2007;68(2):116-21.

11. Wu T, Lv C, Wu L, Chen W, Lv M, Jiang S, et al. Risk of intracranial hemorrhage with direct oral anticoagulants: a systematic review and meta-analysis of randomized controlled trials. J Neurol. 2022;269(2):664-75.
12. DiRisio AC, Harary M, Muskens IS, Yunusa I, Gormley WB, Aglio LS, et al. Outcomes of intraparenchymal hemorrhage after direct oral anticoagulant or vitamin K antagonist therapy: A systematic review and meta-analysis. Journal of Clinical Neuroscience. 2019;62:188-94.
13. Stampfuss J, Kubitza D, Becka M, Mueck W. The effect of food on the absorption and pharmacokinetics of rivaroxaban. Int J Clin Pharmacol Ther. 2013;51(7):549-61.
14. Julia S, James U. Direct oral anticoagulants: A quick guide. Eur Cardiol. 2017;12(1):40-5.
15. Shih AW, Crowther MA. Reversal of direct oral anticoagulants: a practical approach. Hematology Am Soc Hematol Educ Program. 2016;2016(1):612-9.
16. Gosselin RC, Adcock DM, Bates SM, Douxfils J, Favaloro EJ, Gouin-Thibault I, et al. International Council for Standardization in Haematology (ICSH) Recommendations for Laboratory Measurement of Direct Oral Anticoagulants. Thromb Haemost. 2018;118(3):437-50.
17. Dunois C. Laboratory Monitoring of Direct Oral Anticoagulants (DOACs). Biomedicines. 2021;9(5):445.
18. Maguire M, Fuh L, Goldstein JN, Marshall AL, Levine M, Howell ML, et al. Thromboembolic Risk of 4-Factor Prothrombin Complex Concentrate versus Fresh Frozen Plasma for Urgent Warfarin Reversal in the Emergency Department. West J Emerg Med. 2019;20(4):619-25.
19. Chai-Adisaksopha C, Watanabe AH, Dilokthornsakul P, Navaravong L, Witt DM, Chaiyakunapruk N. Impact of type of anticoagulant on clinical outcomes in cancer patients who had atrial fibrillation. Sci Rep. 2023;13(1):10937.
20. Pollack CVJr, Reilly PA, Eikelboom J, Glund S, Verhamme P, Bernstein RA, et al. Idarucizumab for Dabigatran Reversal. New England Journal of Medicine. 2015;373(6):511-20.
21. Horst SFB van der, Martens ESL, Exter PL den, Bos MHA, Mens TE van, Huisman MV, et al. Idarucizumab for dabigatran reversal: A systematic review and meta-analysis of indications and outcomes. Thromb Res. 2023;228:21-32.
22. Siegal DM, Curnutte JT, Connolly SJ, Lu G, Conley PB, Wiens BL, et al. Andexanet Alfa for the Reversal of Factor Xa Inhibitor Activity. N Engl J Med. 2015;373(25):2413-24.
23. Connolly SJ, Sharma M, Cohen AT, Demchuk AM, Członkowska A, Lindgren AG, et al. Andexanet for factor Xa Inhibitor–associated acute intracerebral hemorrhage. N Engl J Med. 2024;390(19):1745-55.
24. Ansell J, Bakhru S, Laulicht BE, Tracey G, Villano S, Freedman D. Ciraparantag reverses the anticoagulant activity of apixaban and rivaroxaban in healthy elderly subjects. Eur Heart J. 2022;43(10):985-92.
25. Shoamanesh A, Mundl H, Smith EE, Masjuan J, Milanov I, Hirano T, et al. Factor XIa inhibition with asundexian after acute non-cardioembolic ischaemic stroke (PACIFIC-Stroke): an international, randomised, double-blind, placebo-controlled, phase 2b trial. Lancet. 2022;400(10357):997-1007.
26. Sharma M, Molina CA, Toyoda K, Bereczki D, Bangdiwala SI, Kasner SE, et al. Safety and efficacy of factor XIa inhibition with milvexian for secondary stroke prevention (AXIOMATIC-SSP): a phase 2, international, randomised, double-blind, placebo-controlled, dose-finding trial. Lancet Neurol. 2024;23(1):46-59.

Aortic Arch Atheroma—Underdiagnosed Stroke Mechanism: Diagnosis and Management

Simerpreet S Bal, Arun Kathuveetil, Diego Antonio Gutierrez Vasquez

ABSTRACT

Atherosclerosis is the most common condition affecting the aortic arch and individuals who have complex aortic atheroma are considered to have high risk for stroke. The question of whether and how to treat these patients is in fact controversial. This review examines the data regarding the classification of aortic plaques, the relationship between atheroma and stroke, the diagnostic imaging, available treatments, and the clinical trials conducted in this clinical scenario.

Keywords: Aortic atheroma, Stroke, Transesophageal echocardiogram, Computed tomography angiography.

■ INTRODUCTION

Aortic atheroma (AA) is a frequent finding in patients with ischemic stroke. But its role as a source of cerebral emboli or a marker of atherosclerosis is unclear. Literature reports a strong association between thoracic AA and risk of stroke, such that significant plaques are seen in up to 14% of patients with a history of stroke and peripheral embolization.[1,2] The most reliable method for detecting AA is transesophageal echocardiogram (TEE); however, computed tomography angiography (CTA) is a reasonable substitute.[3] Other methods, including magnetic resonance imaging (MRI) and positron emission tomography (PET), may also be utilized to assess plaque vulnerability more thoroughly.[3] Despite great interest, it is yet unclear which antithrombotic medication is best, but aggressive lipid-lowering therapy is advised. Based on currently available data, this chapter attempts to provide recommendations for patients with AA regarding diagnosis, treatment, and the causal relationship to stroke **(Figs. 1A to D)**.

■ ANATOMICAL CONSIDERATIONS

The aorta is the largest elastic artery and is classically divided into two anatomical segments—(1) the thoracic aorta and (2) the abdominal aorta. The thoracic aorta includes the aortic root, the ascending tract, the arch, and the descending aorta. The aortic root extends from the annulus to the sinotubular junction (STJ).[4] The ascending aorta comprises the tract from the STJ to approximately the level of the fourth thoracic vertebra, where the brachiocephalic artery takes off. The aortic arch lies between the brachiocephalic artery and the isthmus, distal to the left subclavian artery origin. The descending aorta starts after the takeoff of the left subclavian artery.

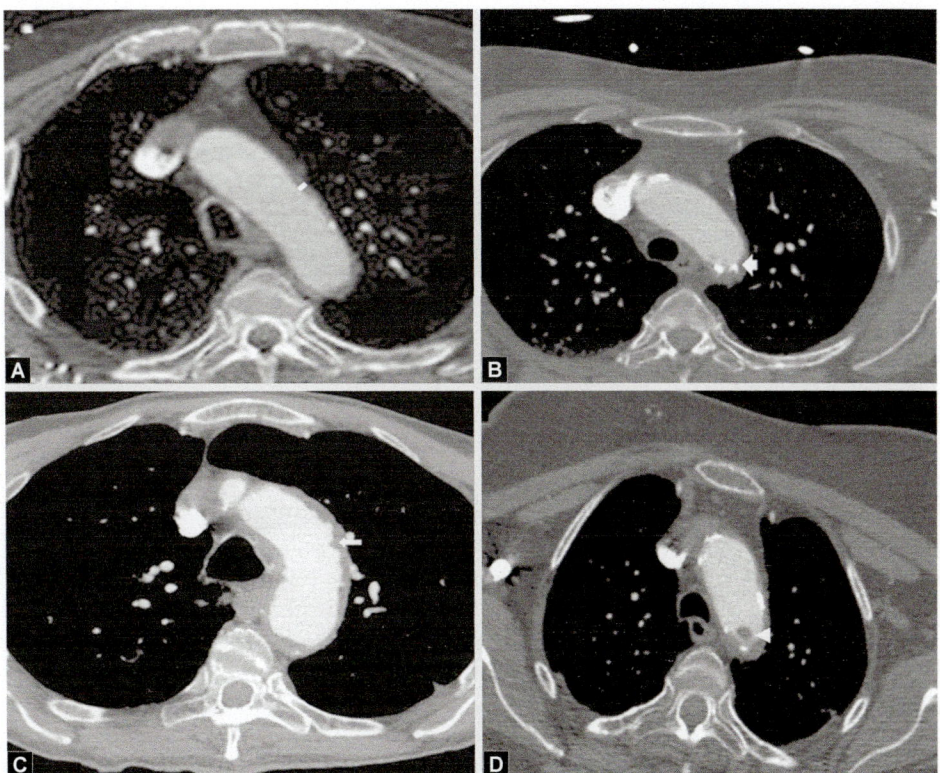

FIGS. 1A TO D: Grading of arch atherosclerosis using CT angiography. (A) Grade 1, 5–10 mm of aortic wall thickness (white line); (B) Grade 2, >10 mm single/multiple areas of linear atheroma with smooth surface (white thick arrow); (C) Grade 3, >10 mm single/multiple areas with irregular surface/ulceration (white long arrow); (D) Grade 4, >10 mm single/multiple complex protruding plaques with neck (white arrowhead).

■ AORTIC ATHEROMA AND EMBOLIC RISK

Aortic atheroma is the most common disease of the aortic arch. Factors that increase the risk of developing AA include age, gender, genetics, high blood pressure, diabetes, high cholesterol, lack of physical activity, tobacco use, and endothelial dysfunction.[5] Factors that increase the risk of embolic complications include inflammation, high blood pressure causing shear forces, plaque bleeding, aneurysm development, and iatrogenic procedures.[5]

Aortic atheroma poses a significant embolic risk when the plaque thickness is ≥4 mm and has a complex morphology.[6,7] Large plaques in the proximal thoracic aorta are a known risk factor for ischemic stroke, with a 2.5- to 9-fold increase in stroke risk in case-control studies and a fourfold increase in prospective studies.[8] AA, regardless of morphology, indicates vascular disease and increases the risk of cerebrovascular events.[9-11] Patients with high-risk AA often have significant carotid lesions, so those with cerebrovascular events and severe carotid disease should have their aortic vessel thoroughly assessed.[8] Results from the French study on Aortic Plaques in Stroke (FAPS) group have provided evidence of a direct relationship between AA and stroke, rather than just an association.[11] The risk of another stroke in individuals with a previous stroke history and large or complex AA has shown to be consistently high.[6] Extensive plaques in the aortic arch show a clear potential to cause embolisms, as evidenced by the frequent microembolic signals detected during transcranial Doppler.[12] Additionally, it has been demonstrated by the FAPS that patients with severe AA have a high risk of stroke within 1 year.[11] The occurrence of perioperative stroke following cardiac surgery and percutaneous procedures is a serious complication, with a reported incidence ranging from 2 to 3% in general surgical patients, and potential to increase up to 7% in high-risk elderly individuals with protruding AA.[13]

While AA located in the ascending aorta and proximal aortic arch may embolize to the brain through supra-aortic vessels by anterograde flow,[14] plaques located in the descending thoracic aorta can still be involved in embolism.[15,16] Recent studies showed that retrograde flow from the proximal descending aorta is very common and it mainly reached to the left subclavian artery (98%), but the diastolic blood flow reversal is also visualized in the left common carotid artery (42.1%) and even in the brachiocephalic trunk (31.0%).[17] The most common pattern of ischemic lesions in patients with vulnerable AA is the presence of multiple small cortical lesions in multiple vascular territories, including the posterior circulation.[18,19] Nevertheless, the presence of a single small subcortical lesion is not uncommon.[20]

DIAGNOSIS

Echocardiography

Transesophageal Echocardiography

The TEE, invented in the 1970s, offers high-resolution images of the whole thoracic aorta except for a tiny portion of the ascending aorta and origin of innominate artery, which is obscured by the tracheal air column.[21] TEE is the recommended method for identifying, quantifying, and characterizing thoracic AA.[22] It can be used to evaluate the thickness of an intimal plaque, ulcerations, calcifications, and superimposed mobile thrombi.[22] Though transthoracic echocardiography (TTE) can be used to visualize the AA, its resolution is poor than that of the images obtained by TEE. Intravascular ultrasound in conjunction with TTE can produce higher quality images. But it could result in iatrogenic embolization and is too invasive to be employed as a routine diagnostic tool for AA.[23] The following plaque characteristics are assessed using TEE:

- *Plaque thickness*: The normal aorta has a smooth intimal surface with a thickness of ≤1 mm on TEE.[22] AA leads to intimal thickening because of the migration of smooth muscle cells and foam cells from the media associated with calcification and ulceration. Katz et al. suggested a five-point grading system **(Table 1)** for the plaques and assessed the incidence of stroke.[13] TEE was utilized by the FAPS investigators to assess the thickness of the AA in a subset of stroke patients.[2] They observed that patients with a plaque thickness of ≥4 mm had a considerably higher odds ratio (OR) for stroke and

TABLE 1: Grading of aortic atheroma.[13]

Grade	Description	Percentage of incidence of stroke
1	Normal aorta	0
2	Extensive intimal thickness < 3 mm	0
3	Protrudes < 5 mm into the lumen	5
4	Protrudes > 5 mm into the lumen	10.5
5	Mobile atheroma	46.5

that increasing plaque thickness was associated with an increased risk. For plaques ranging in thickness from 1 to 3.9 mm, the OR was 3.9, and for plaques ≥4 mm, it was 13.8 **(Figs. 2A to D)**.[24]
- *Plaque morphology and plaque thrombosis (Figs. 3A to C)*:
  ○ *Ulceration*: In 1992, a seminal autopsy investigation looked at thoracic aorta of 500 patients who had suffered from stroke and other neurologic conditions, and it was observed that ulcerated plaques were present in the aortic arch of 26% of patients with stroke. AAs were present in 61% of patients with cryptogenic stroke. There is a greater risk of stroke for ulcerations ≥ 2 mm. These ulcerations were observed in 8% of patients with stroke of determined etiology, 7% of individuals without stroke, and 39% of patients with cryptogenic stroke.[25]
  ○ *Calcification*: Despite the fact that calcification is one sign of the atherosclerotic process, large high-risk plaques frequently lack calcification.[13] The FAPS investigators examined the plaque morphology of 334 stroke patients > 60 years using TEE and observed that plaques with thickness ≥ 4 mm were associated with a higher risk of developing ulcers, calcification, and hypoechoic regions. Remarkably, the highest stroke risk was seen in plaques which lack calcification (OR 10.3).[26]
  ○ *Mobile thrombus*: The capacity to image high-risk mobile components which are thought to depict superimposed thrombi is one of the benefits

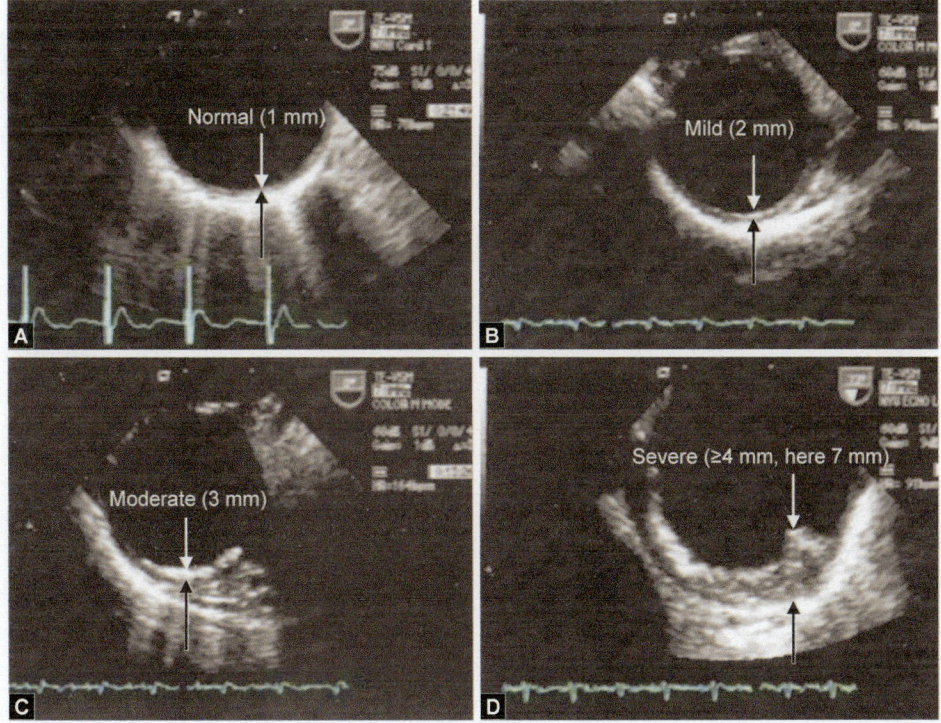

FIGS. 2A TO D: Transesophageal echocardiography showing normal aortic intima (1 mm) and mild (2 mm), moderate (3 mm), and severe (≥4 mm; shown here = 7 mm) plaque.

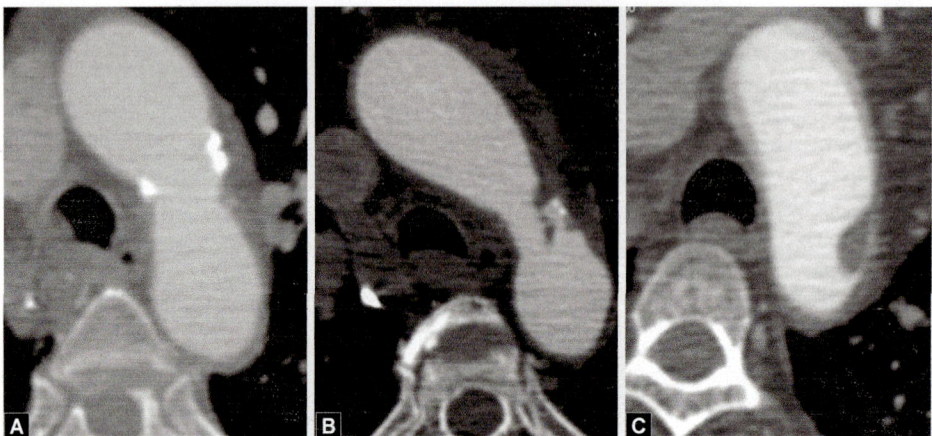

FIGS. 3A TO C: Axial CT angiogram of aortic arch showing plaques of varying morphology—(A) Plaque > 4 mm thick. (B) Ulcerated plaque over the anterior wall of aorta; (C) Protruding plaque over the anterolateral wall of aorta.

of TEE.[27] Embolization of thrombus from AA has been demonstrated with the specimens extracted from femoral arteries of patients with acute limb ischemia which highlights that these mobile components have significant embolic risk. Similarly, cerebral embolism of thrombus resulting from AA may contribute to stroke.[9]

o *Protruding plaques*: Up to one-third of patients with a protruding AA is likely to experience vascular events within a year.[28] Although the best treatment with a protruding AA is still not fully established, it is crucial to fully evaluate the patient's aortic condition prior to any catheterization or open-heart surgery because these patients are highly susceptible to embolization. Moreover, when these patients received heparin or coumadin treatment, there was a regression of superimposed thrombi on TEE.[29]

For the diagnosis of mobile thrombi and measurement of plaque thickness, the majority of echocardiographers believe that TEE is more accurate than TTE. TEE probe is positioned closer to the aorta and can operate at a higher frequency. TEE is safe, may be used at the patient's bedside. It is feasible to accurately and thoroughly evaluate the aorta, including the origin of the great vessels. The main drawbacks of TEE include patient discomfort of gagging, need to use conscious sedation and rare possibility of esophageal and oropharyngeal injury. Approximately, 2% of the plaques may go unnoticed due to the "blind spot" created by tracheal air column.[28]

TEE—"A" View Method

The distal ascending aorta and aortic arch can be examined using the recently developed A-view approach, a variation of traditional TEE. This method was developed to overcome the "blind spot" created by the air-filled trachea. This technique replaces the air in the distal trachea and left main bronchus with an intratracheal balloon filled with saline.[30]

Epiaortic Ultrasound

In order to directly see the aortic valve and its function during surgery, epiaortic ultrasound (EAU) was first employed in the 1970s.[31] Over the years, its application extended to AA as well. EAU is the conventional "gold standard" for detecting intraoperative AA. The transducer is positioned directly on the aorta during the procedure, following the sternotomy which enables a better acoustic window and better identification of plaques, with a lower risk of embolization.[32] Moreover, EAU appears to be more sensitive than TEE and there is "no blind spot". It is advised to use EAU while performing surgery on the ascending aorta and if an AA of >3 mm thickness is detected, manual palpation should be avoided.[33]

Computed Tomography Angiography (Figs. 4A and B)

Another diagnostic modality that highlights the aortic lumen with contrast is computed tomography angiography (CTA). With the advent of CTA, the sensitivity, specificity, and accuracy for detecting AA approach higher than that of TEE.[22] It is a noninvasive method which can be utilized for assessing the progression and regression of AA.[34] Tenenbaum et al. evaluated calcium deposits and hypoattenuation along the aortic wall using unenhanced CT in patients with recent stroke and they discovered that selecting a threshold of 4-mm thickness for AA produced the greatest results in terms of sensitivity (87%) and specificity (82%).[35] This is in excellent agreement with the 4-mm threshold observed in the FAPS for predicting a markedly elevated risk of stroke.[25]

Within the vessel wall (VW), lipid-rich or fibrous plaque manifests as hypoattenuated dark signals, while calcified plaque

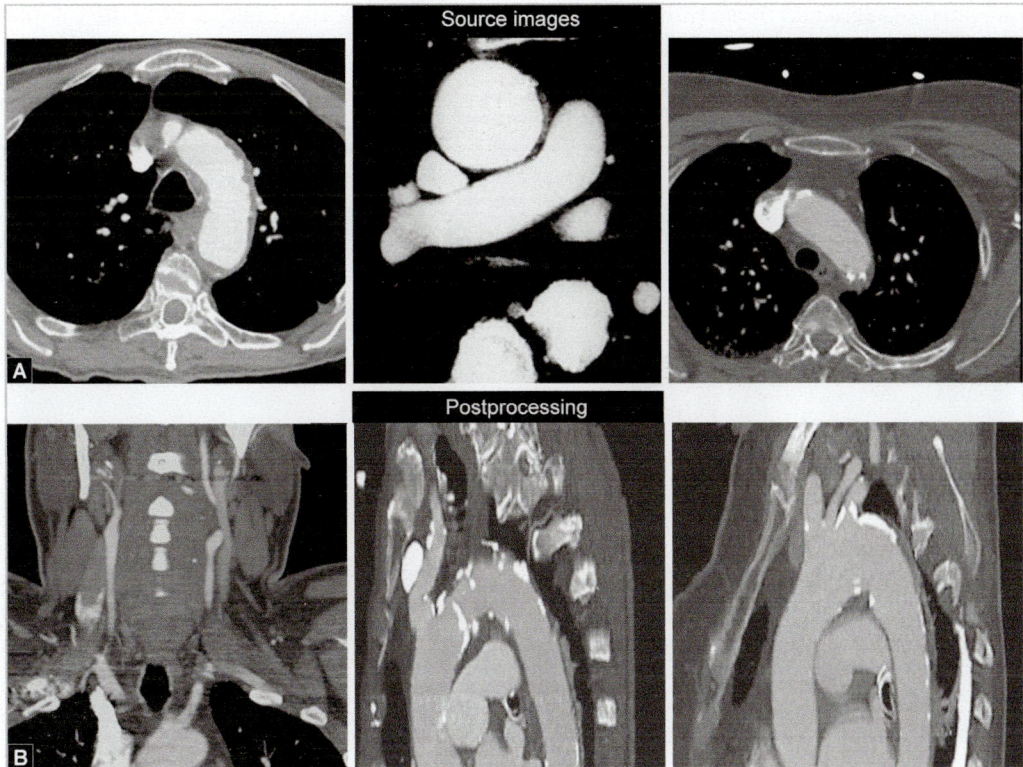

FIGS. 4A AND B: (A) CTA source images (top) showing aortic arch atherosclerosis and postprocessing (B) CTA images (bottom) showing extent of aortic arch atherosclerosis.

appears as a light, high-attenuation signal.[35] A subgroup analysis of NAVIGATE ESUS defined AA as complex, when the thickness ≥ 4 mm, ulcerated, or were mobile and they were associated with 8% increased risk of stroke.[36] Another study defined aortic plaques characteristics as (1) large aortic plaque, as fixed plaque ≥ 4 mm in thickness, (2) ulceration, as plaque which appears like a crater that was >2 mm in depth and width, and (3) protruding plaque, as plaque components that protrude freely into the aortic lumen. The complex plaque included large plaques with ulceration and/or protruding components.[37] To conclude, there are no large CTA data to classify which aortic plaque is clinically significant leading to recurrent stroke. However, there is consensus that plaques thickness ≥ 4 mm increases the risk of recurrent strokes. Furthermore, ulcerated plaques and those with protruding components have been shown to increase the stroke risk.

The CTA has the potential to be advantageous since it can continuously image the entire aorta, something that TEE cannot do. In the aortic arch, CTA could detect four times as many plaques as TEE. This allows for a semiquantitative assessment of the aortic plaque burden.[38] The main drawbacks of CTA include the need for contrast agents, comparatively high radiation dosage, unable to use in the operating room during cardiac surgery and inability to demonstrate the mobility of the plaques.[38]

Magnetic Resonance Imaging (Figs. 5A to C)

Magnetic resonance imaging has been shown to be a reliable tool for evaluating the structure and composition of plaque

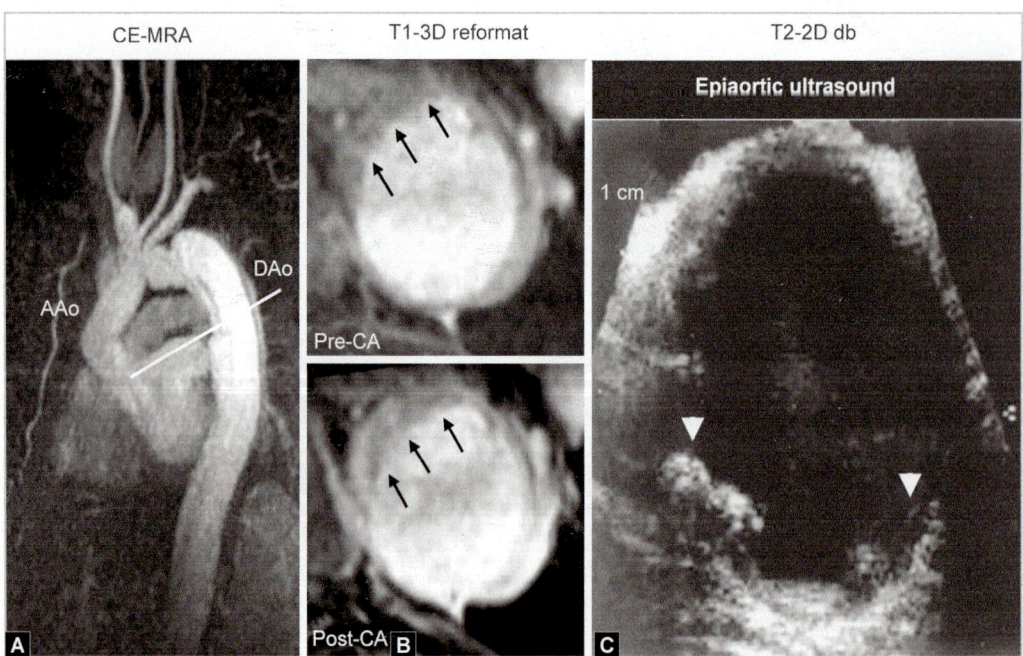

FIGS. 5A TO C: Contrast-enhanced magnetic resonance angiogram (CE MRA) showing plaques in the ascending and descending aorta, T1 3D reformat MRI (pre- and postcontrast) showing circumferential plaques in the aorta (black arrows), epiaortic ultrasound showing plaque in the aorta (white arrowheads).

in both human and experimental models of atherosclerosis. Plaque progression and regression can be monitored using MRI due to its high resolution.[39] 3T MRI showed more promising results when compared with 1.5T MRI and TEE.[40,41] Image acquisition includes three-dimensional (3D) magnetic resonance-time of flight (MR TOF) angiography; T1-weighted pre- and postcontrast spin echo [T1-weighted imaging (T1WI)] or a double inversion recovery technique, T2-weighted spin echo imaging (T2WI) and T1W fat saturated spin echo imaging. The components of the plaque can be intracellular lipid and extracellular lipid core, loose connective tissue/collagen matrix/fibrocellular, calcifications, and hemorrhagic components **(Table 2)**. High-resolution MRI can visualize fibrous cap and focal ulcers and differentiate fibrocellular components from the lipid core or hemorrhagic components using a multispectral approach.[42]

Magnetic resonance imaging detect complex plaques more than TEE at the aortic arch but potentially overestimated the wall thickness.[43] Regarding its capacity to identify ulceration, 3D MRI has shown conflicting results when directly compared to TEE.[44] Electrocardiography (ECG)-gated cine imaging, a form of MRI sequence to capture motion has been recently developed to identify mobile thrombus.[43] In these studies, structures within the blood stream that were mobile on CINE imaging were defined as mobile thrombus.[44] Aortic VW-MRI has been utilized to look at the compositions of plaques. 3T MRI using a T1W MPRAGE fat suppressed pulse sequence is used to evaluate vulnerable plaques.[45] The liver acquisition with volume acceleration-flexible (LAVA-Flex) technique was used by Morihara et al. to evaluate the correlation between the thickness of the plaque on TEE and high-intensity plaque lesions in AA. Approximately, 87.5% of the hyperintense aortic lesions showed a ≥4-mm plaque on TEE, which was considered the gold standard. With patients who had significant aortic plaques (thickness ≥ 4), LAVA-Flex demonstrated a sensitivity of 95.5% and a specificity of 88.0%.[46] 4D flow MRI can be used to analyze hemodynamic flow parameters and look at aortic wall thickness and stiffness as well as flow reversal in the proximal descending aorta.[47] These cutting-edge imaging methods are currently potential research tools and may find use in the assessment of AA in the future.

There are both advantages and limitations to MRI of aortic atherosclerosis when compared with TEE and CT **(Table 3)**. Both MRI and CT are less invasive than TEE and can evaluate the entire aorta. Like CT, MRI

TABLE 2: Plaque components on various imaging sequences.

Plaque components	T2WI	T1WI	MR TOF	Postcontrast T1WI
Recent hemorrhage	Variable	High-to-moderate (high with FS)	High	No
Lipid-rich core	Variable (low, typically)	High (low with FS)	Moderate	No
Hydrophilic necrosis	Very high	Low	Low	No
Fibrous tissue	Variable (moderate, typically)	Moderate	Moderate-to-low	Yes
Calcification	Low	Low	Low	No

(FS: fat saturated; MR TOF: magnetic resonance-time of flight)

Source: Adapted from Choe YH. Noninvasive Imaging od atherosclerotic plaques using MRI and CT. Korean Circ J. 2005;35:1-14.

has limitations when it comes to identifying mobile components and thrombi, which are easily seen on TEE. These limitations, however, may be overcome with new MRI techniques.[48]

Positron Emission Tomography–Computed Tomography

By using fluorine 18 (18F) fluorodeoxyglucose (FDG) as a glucose analogue in PET, it is possible to identify areas with active atherosclerotic change by detecting increased tissue uptake of glucose. The accumulation of FDG in the aortic wall has been linked to subendothelial smooth muscle growth and a notable cellular infiltration inside active atherosclerotic plaques.[49] By fusing PET and CT images, it is possible to determine high-risk susceptible plaques and to assess the location, distribution, and degree of active atherosclerosis. The clinical efficacy of PET/CT for imaging AA is still unknown.[49]

■ TREATMENT

Medical Management

Antithrombotic Treatment

The best antithrombotic therapy for patients with AA is still not clear. Various antithrombotic approaches which include aspirin, combination of antiplatelets, warfarin, and combination of low-dose warfarin with aspirin have been tried. Retrospective studies demonstrated a possible advantage of warfarin compared to aspirin.[50,51] Nevertheless, these findings were not substantiated in comparative control trials or in clinical research.[36,52,53]

There has been only one prospective randomized trial conducted specifically in patients with AA and stroke. The Aortic Arch Related Cerebral Hazard Trial (ARCH) study looked at whether aspirin plus clopidogrel (A + C) was better than warfarin with a target INR of 2.5 in patients with ischemic stroke, transient ischemic attack (TIA), or peripheral embolism, and AA > 4 mm. The study included 349 participants for over 8 years and was terminated prematurely. In the study, 7.6% of those taking A + C and 11.3% of those on warfarin experienced cardiovascular events, vascular death, or intracranial hemorrhage. Nevertheless, this difference was not statistically significant.[52]

A subset of Warfarin and Aspirin for the Prevention of Recurrent Ischemic Stroke study (WARSS) patients increased risk of stroke recurrence or death when having larger AA (26.7%), in comparison to those with no plaques (10%) or small ones (16.5%).[56] They conducted a comparison between aspirin 325 mg and warfarin, determining that the risk was equal for both treatments (aspirin 15.8% vs. warfarin 16.4%, $p = 0.43$), even for patients with large plaques.[54] A subgroup analysis of NAVIGATE ESUS compared the use of aspirin 100 mg and rivaroxaban 15 mg in patients with AA and observed no difference in annual risk of stroke recurrence in patients with complex and noncomplex plaques. A recent meta-analysis including these three previous trials found no difference for treatment with anticoagulation versus antiplatelet in AA (OR 0.80; 95% CI 0.40–1.62).[53]

In summary, the effectiveness of antithrombotic treatment in preventing stroke or recurrence in AA patients is still not confirmed, with a single antiplatelet therapy being the preferred approach as advised in atherosclerotic cardiovascular disease guidelines. If there is a mobile blood clot, short-term use of anticoagulants may be appropriate for specific situations.

Hyperlipidemia

In the Treat Stroke to Target (TST) trial, patients with prior stroke or atherosclerosis, including TIA and AA, were treated with statins and/or ezetimibe to achieve LDL levels of 100 versus < 70 mg/dL. Levels < 70 mg/dL showed a reduction in cardiovascular events

TABLE 3: Comparison of various diagnostic modalities in the evaluation of AA.

Modality	Advantages	Disadvantages
Transesophageal echocardiography	• Widely used, easy availability, low cost • Highly reproducible • Detect plaque size and mobility • Free of ionizing radiation and contrast exposure • High resolution of aortic intima and lumen interface	• Limited visualization of distal ascending aorta and proximal arch • Plaque composition cannot be determined
Computed axial tomography angiogram	• Sensitive, specific, noninvasive, and accurate • Assess the entire aorta, plaque burden and characteristics	• Exposure to radiation and contrast • Limited utility in assessing mobile plaque • Expensive
Magnetic resonance imaging	• Assess entire aortic arch, plaque composition and stability • Noninvasive	• Expensive, limited availability • Spatial resolution is inferior to computed axial tomogram • Overestimates plaque thickness • Contraindicated with ferromagnetic implants and pacemakers • Claustrophobia
Epiaortic echocardiography	Better resolution and superior to TEE in detecting AA in operating room	• Not routinely used • Requires technical expertise

(AA: aortic atheroma; TEE: transesophageal echocardiogram)

recurrence or death.[55] In a retrospective match-paired study for 12 years and there was 12% reduction in clinical events in patients on statins compared to 29% on nonstatin patients.[56] Although the key goal seems to be a low LDL-C rather than a specific drug, there is documentation of stabilization of aortic plaques with rosuvastatin in the EPISTEME trial, that showed an significant increment in the proportion of high-echoic plaque and a decrease of low-echoic areas seen in TEE after treatment with rosuvastatin 5 mg for 6 months, while the control group saw a decrease of high-echoic plaque areas. This may suggest that rosuvastatin might stabilize the atherosclerotic plaque by reducing its lipid-rich necrotic core and increasing its collagen structure.[57] Likewise, the observations of the RAPID study using serial MR showed a greater regression in thoracic aortic plaques at 1 year of therapy with a more intense low-density lipoprotein cholesterol (LDL-C) lowering and higher doses of rosuvastatin.[58]

Interventional Treatment

Endovascular treatment not only removes the thrombus but also treats the underlying cause by covering the atherosclerotic aortic wall.[59] Endovascular stent graft repair is a novel, safe, and effective therapeutic option for patients with penetrating atherosclerotic ulcer (PAU), but there is a limited experience in preventing aortic rupture or aneurysm formation in the long-term course.[60] Currently, there is insufficient evidence to recommend prophylactic aortic arch stenting for purposes of stroke prevention.

Surgical Treatment

Aortic arch endarterectomy has been attempted for patients with thromboembolism originating from aortic arch atheroma. Although successful in a handful of case reports, this procedure resulted in a relatively high rate (34.9% with endarterectomy vs. 11.6% without endarterectomy) of perioperative stroke and mortality when it was performed to limit stroke during cardiac surgical procedures.[61] Clearly, the role of surgery, in the presence of high-risk aortic plaques, is still controversial; and prospective, randomized clinical study comparing surgery versus medical therapy will be mandatory to provide conclusive evidence in this respect.

CONCLUSION

The question whether AA is a risk factor, or an innocent bystander seems to remain unanswered, but patients with complicated AA should be considered at risk for stroke. We suggest AA visualization in the workup of patients with ischemic stroke as it may alter the preventive treatment.

REFERENCES

1. Agmon Y, Khandheria BK, Meissner I, Schwartz GL, Petterson TM, O'Fallon WM, et al. Independent association of high blood pressure and aortic atherosclerosis. Circulation. 2000;102(17):2087-93.
2. Amarenco P, Cohen A, Tzourio C, Bertrand B, Hommel M, Besson G, et al. Atherosclerotic disease of the aortic arch and the risk of ischemic stroke. N Engl J Med. 1994;331(22):1474-9.
3. Viedma-Guiard E, Guidoux C, Amarenco P, Meseguer E. Aortic sources of embolism. Front Neurol. 2021;11:606663.
4. di Gioia CRT, Ascione A, Carletti R, Giordano C. Thoracic aorta: Anatomy and pathology. Diagnostics. 2023;13(13):2166.
5. Vizzardi E, Gelsomino S, D'Aloia A, Lorusso R. Aortic atheromas and stroke: Review of literature. J Investig Med. 2013;61(6):956-66.
6. Macleod MR, Amarenco P, Davis SM, Donnan GA. Aortic arch atheroma and the risk of stroke Atheroma of the aortic arch: an important and poorly recognised factor in the aetiology of stroke. Lancet Neurol. 2004;3(July):408-14.
7. Jones EF, Kalman JM, Calafiore P, Tonkin AM, Donnan GA. Proximal aortic atheroma. An independent risk factor for cerebral ischemia. Stroke. 1995;26(2):218-24.
8. Thenappan T, Ali Raza J, Movahed A. Aortic atheromas: Current concepts and controversies—A review of the literature. Echocardiography. 2008;25(2):198-207.
9. Tullio MR Di, Russo C, Jin Z, Sacco RL, Mohr JP, Homma S, et al. Aortic arch plaques and risk of recurrent stroke and death. Circulation. 2009;119:2376-83.
10. Fujimoto S, Yasaka M, Otsubo R, Oe H, Nagatsuka K, Minematsu K. Aortic arch atherosclerotic lesions and the recurrence of ischemic stroke. Stroke. 2004;35(6):1426-9.
11. Cohen A, Tzourio C, Bertrand B, Chauvel C, Bousser MG, Amarenco P. Aortic plaque morphology and vascular events a follow-up study in patients with ischemic stroke. Circulation. 1997;96:3838-41.
12. Castellanos M, Serena J, Segura T, Pérez-Ayuso MJ, Silva Y, Dávalos A. Atherosclerotic aortic arch plaques in cryptogenic stroke: A microembolic signal monitoring study. Eur Neurol. 2001;45(3):145-50.
13. Katz ES, Tunick PA, Rusinek H, Ribakove G, Spencer FC, Kronzon I. Protruding aortic atheromas predict stroke in elderly patients undergoing cardiopulmonary bypass: Experience with intraoperative transesophageal echocardiography. J Am Coll Cardiol. 1992;20(1):70-7.
14. Viguier A, Pavy le Traon A, Massabuau P, Valton L, Larrue V. Asymptomatic cerebral embolic signals in patients with acute cerebral ischaemia and severe aortic arch atherosclerosis. J Neurol. 2001;248(9):768-71.
15. Harloff A, Simon J, Brendecke S, Assefa D, Helbing T, Frydrychowicz A, et al. Complex plaques in the proximal descending aorta. Stroke. 2010;41(6):1145-50.
16. Katsanos AH, Giannopoulos S, Kosmidou M, Voumvourakis K, Parissis JT, Kyritsis AP, et al. Complex atheromatous plaques in the descending aorta and the risk of stroke. Stroke. 2014;45(6):1764-70.

17. Harloff A, Hagenlocher P, Lodemann T, Hennemuth A, Weiller C, Hennig J, et al. Retrograde aortic blood flow as a mechanism of stroke: MR evaluation of the prevalence in a population-based study. Eur Radiol. 2019;29(10):5172-9.
18. Kim SJ, Ryoo S, Hwang J, Noh HJ, Park JH, Choe YH, et al. Characterization of the infarct pattern caused by vulnerable aortic arch atheroma: DWI and multidetector row CT study. Cerebrovasc Dis. 2012;33(6):549-57.
19. Shimada JI, Yasaka M, Wakugawa Y, Ogata T, Makihara N, Ito S, et al. Features of brain magnetic resonance imaging diffusion-weighted images of aortogenic embolic stroke. Circ J. 2014;78(3):738-42.
20. Kim SW, Kim YD, Chang HJ, Hong GR, Shim CY, Chung SJ, et al. Different infarction patterns in patients with aortic atheroma compared to those with cardioembolism or large artery atherosclerosis. J Neurol. 2018;265(1):151-8.
21. Frazin L, Talano JV, Stephanides L, Loeb HS, Kopel L, Gunnar RM. Esophageal echocardiography. Circulation. 1976;54(1):102-8.
22. Tunick PA, Krinsky GA, Lee VS, Kronzon I. Diagnostic imaging of thoracic aortic atherosclerosis. Am J Roentgenol. 2000;174(4):1119-25.
23. Williams DM, Lee DY, Hamilton BH, Marx MV, Narasimham DL, Kazanjian SN, et al. The dissected aorta: part III. Anatomy and radiologic diagnosis of branch-vessel compromise. Radiology. 1997;203(1):37-44.
24. French Study of Aortic Plaques in Stroke Group; Amerenco P, Cohen A, Hommel M, Moulin T, Leys D, Bousser MG. Atherosclerotic disease of the aortic arch as a risk factor for recurrent ischemic stroke. N Engl J Med. 1996;334:1216-21.
25. Amarengo P, Duyckaerts C, Tzourio C, Hénin D, Bousser MG, Hauw JJ. The prevalence of ulcerated plaques in the aortic arch in patients with stroke. N Engl J Med. 1992;326(4):221-5.
26. Cohen A, Tzourio C, Bertrand B, Chauvel C, Bousser MG, Amarenco P. Aortic plaque morphology and vascular events. Circulation. 1997;96(11):3838-41.
27. Tunick PA, Rosenzweig BP, Katz ES, Freedberg RS, Perez JL, Kronzon I. High risk for vascular events in patients with protruding aortic atheromas: A prospective study. J Am Coll Cardiol. 1994;23(5):1085-90.
28. Kronzon I, Tunick PA. Aortic atherosclerotic disease and stroke. Circulation. 2006;114(1):63-75.
29. Krinsky GA, Freedberg R, Lee VS, Rockman C, Tunick PA. Innominate artery atheroma: A lesion seen with gadolinium-enhanced MR angiography and often missed by transesophageal echocardiography. Clin Imaging. 2001;25(4):251-7.
30. Patil TA, Nierich A. Transesophageal echocardiography evaluation of the thoracic aorta. Ann Card Anaesth. 2016;19(Supplement):S44-55.
31. Niklewski T, Zembala M, Puszczewicz D, Nadziakiewicz P, Karolak W, Zembala M. The use of intraoperative epiaortic ultrasonography in monitoring patients over 75 years old treated with aortic valve replacement. Kardiochir Torakochirurgia Pol. 2017;14(1):10-5.
32. Suvarna S, Smith A, Stygall J, Kolvecar S, Walesby R, Harrison M, et al. An intraoperative assessment of the ascending aorta: a comparison of digital palpation, transesophageal echocardiography, and epiaortic ultrasonography. J Cardiothorac Vasc Anesth. 2007;21(6):805-9.
33. Glas KE, Swaminathan M, Reeves ST, Shanewise JS, Rubenson D, Smith PK, et al. Guidelines for the performance of a comprehensive intraoperative epiaortic ultrasonographic examination: Recommendations of the American Society of Echocardiography and the Society of Cardiovascular Anesthesiologists; Endorsed by the Society of Thoracic Surgeons. J Am Soc Echocardiogr. 2007;20(11):1227-35.
34. Takasu J, Masuda Y, Watanabe S, Funabashi N, Aoyagi Y, Onishi M, et al. Progression and regression of atherosclerotic findings in the descending thoracic aorta detected by enhanced computed tomography. Atherosclerosis. 1994;110(2):175-84.
35. Tenenbaum A, Garniek A, Shemesh J, Fisman EZ, Stroh CI, Itzchak Y, et al. Dual-helical CT for detecting aortic atheromas as a source of stroke: comparison with transesophageal echocardiography. Radiology. 1998;208(1):153-8.
36. Ntaios G, Pearce LA, Meseguer E, Endres M, Amarenco P, Ozturk S, et al. Aortic arch atherosclerosis in patients with embolic stroke of undetermined source. Stroke. 2019;50(11):3184-90.
37. Arun K, Nambiar P, Kannath S, Sreedharan S, Sukumaran S, Sarma S, et al. Prevalence of aortic plaques in cryptogenic ischemic stroke: Correlation to vascular risk factors and future events. Neurol India. 2022;70(1):182.
38. Boyko M, Chaturvedi S, Beland B, Najm M, Demchuk AM, Menon BK, et al. Prevalence of high-risk aortic arch atherosclerosis features on computed tomography angiography in embolic stroke of undetermined source. J Stroke Cerebrovasc Dis. 2023;32(12):107374.
39. Wehrum T, Dragonu I, Strecker C, Hennig J, Harloff A. Multi-contrast and three-dimensional assessment of the aortic wall using 3 T MRI. Eur J Radiol. 2017;91:148-54.

40. Kutz SM, Lee VS, Tunick PA, Krinsky GA, Kronzon I. Atheromas of the thoracic aorta: A comparison of transesophageal echocardiography and breath-hold gadolinium-enhanced 3-dimensional magnetic resonance angiography. J Am Soc Echocardiogr. 1999;12(10):853-8.
41. Fayad ZA, Nahar T, Fallon JT, Goldman M, Aguinaldo JG, Badimon JJ, et al. In vivo magnetic resonance evaluation of atherosclerotic plaques in the human thoracic aorta. Circulation. 2000;101(21):2503-9.
42. Serfaty JM, Chaabane L, Tabib A, Chevallier JM, Briguet A, Douek PC. Atherosclerotic plaques: Classification and characterization with T2-weighted high-spatial-resolution MR imaging—An in vitro study. Radiology. 2001;219(2):403-10.
43. Harloff A, Dudler P, Frydrychowicz A, Strecker C, Stroh AL, Geibel A, et al. Reliability of aortic MRI at 3 Tesla in patients with acute cryptogenic stroke. J Neurol Neurosurg Psychiatry. 2008;79(5):540-6.
44. Harloff A, Brendecke SM, Simon J, Assefa D, Wallis W, Helbing T, et al. 3D MRI provides improved visualization and detection of aortic arch plaques compared to transesophageal echocardiography. J Magn Reson Imaging. 2012;36(3):604-11.
45. Yamaguchi Y, Tanaka T, Morita Y, Yoshimura S, Koga M, Ihara M, et al. Associations of high intensities on magnetization-prepared rapid acquisition with gradient echo with aortic complicated lesions in ischemic stroke patients. Cerebrovasc Dis. 2019;47(1-2):15-23.
46. Morihara K, Nakano T, Mori K, Fukui I, Nomura M, Suzuki K, et al. Usefulness of rapid MR angiography using two-point Dixon for evaluating carotid and aortic plaques. Neuroradiology. 2022;64(4):693-702.
47. Jarvis K, Soulat G, Scott M, Vali A, Pathrose A, Syed AA, et al. Investigation of aortic wall thickness, stiffness and flow reversal in patients with cryptogenic stroke: A <scp>4D</scp> Flow <scp>MRI</scp> Study. J Magn Reson Imaging. 2021;53(3):942-52.
48. Corti R. Noninvasive imaging of atherosclerotic vessels by MRI for clinical assessment of the effectiveness of therapy. Pharmacol Ther. 2006;110(1):57-70.
49. Tatsumi M, Cohade C, Nakamoto Y, Wahl RL. Fluorodeoxyglucose uptake in the aortic wall at PET/CT: Possible finding for active atherosclerosis. Radiology. 2003;229(3):831-7.
50. Ferrari E, Vidal R, Chevallier T, Baudouy M. Atherosclerosis of the thoracic aorta and aortic debris as a marker of poor prognosis: Benefit of oral anticoagulants. J Am Coll Cardiol. 1999;33(5):1317-22.
51. Dressler FA, Craig WR, Castello R, Labovitz AJ. Mobile aortic atheroma and systemic emboli: Efficacy of anticoagulation and influence of plaque morphology on recurrent stroke. J Am Coll Cardiol. 1998;31(1):134-8.
52. Amarenco P, Davis S, Jones EF, Cohen AA, Heiss WD, Kaste M, et al. Clopidogrel plus aspirin versus warfarin in patients with stroke and aortic arch plaques. Stroke. 2014;45(5):1248-57.
53. Kasner SE, Swaminathan B, Lavados P, Sharma M, Muir K, Veltkamp R, et al. Rivaroxaban or aspirin for patent foramen ovale and embolic stroke of undetermined source: A prespecified subgroup analysis from the NAVIGATE ESUS trial. Lancet Neurol. 2018;17(12):1053-60.
54. Mohr JP, Thompson JLP, Lazar RM, Levin B, Sacco RL, Furie KL, et al. A Comparison of warfarin and aspirin for the prevention of recurrent ischemic stroke. N Engl J Med. 2001;345(20):1444-51.
55. Amarenco P, Kim JS, Labreuche J, Charles H, Abtan J, Béjot Y, et al. A Comparison of two LDL cholesterol targets after ischemic stroke. N Engl J Med. 2020;382(1):9-19.
56. Tunick PA, Nayar AC, Goodkin GM, Mirchandani S, Francescone S, Rosenzweig BP, et al. Effect of treatment on the incidence of stroke and other emboli in 519 patients with severe thoracic aortic plaque. Am J Cardiol. 2002;90(12):1320-5.
57. Ueno Y, Yamashiro K, Tanaka Y, Watanabe M, Miyamoto N, Shimada Y, et al. Rosuvastatin may stabilize atherosclerotic aortic plaque: Transesophageal echocardiographic study in the EPISTEME trial. Atherosclerosis. 2015;239(2):476-82.
58. Yogo M, Sasaki M, Ayaori M, Kihara T, Sato H, Takiguchi S, et al. Intensive lipid lowering therapy with titrated rosuvastatin yields greater atherosclerotic aortic plaque regression: Serial magnetic resonance imaging observations from RAPID study. Atherosclerosis. 2014;232(1):31-9.
59. Criado E, Wall P, Lucas P, Gasparis A, Proffit T, Ricotta J. Transesophageal echo-guided endovascular exclusion of thoracic aortic mobile thrombi. J Vasc Surg. 2004;39(1):238-42.
60. Eggebrecht H, Baumgart D, Schmermund A, von Birgelen C, Herold U, Wiesemes R, et al. Endovascular Stent-graft repair for penetrating atherosclerotic ulcer of the descending aorta. Am J Cardiol. 2003;91(9):1150-3.
61. Muehrcke DD, Grimm RA, Niessen SE, Cosgrove DM. Recurrent cerebral vascular accidents are an indication for ascending aortic endarterectomy. Ann Thorac Surg. 1996;61(5):1516-8.

Recent Advances in the Management of Cerebral Venous Thrombosis

Debjyoti Dhar, TA Sangeeth, MM Samim, Sanjith Aaron, Girish Baburao Kulkarni

ABSTRACT

Cerebral venous thrombosis (CVT) represents 0.5–3% of all strokes, predominantly affecting young individuals, women of reproductive age, and those with a prothrombotic state. The clinical presentation of CVT is varied, including headaches and seizures, necessitating a high index of clinical suspicion for diagnosis. Diagnostic tools primarily include magnetic resonance imaging/magnetic resonance venography (MRI/MRV) or computed tomography/computed tomographic venography (CT/CTV). The clinical trajectory of CVT can be unpredictable, with 10–15% of patients experiencing death or dependence despite intensive medical treatment. This review is based on the latest guidelines laid down by American Heart Association/American Stroke Association (AHA/ASA) 2024 for diagnosing and managing CVT. It emphasizes advancements in diagnostic methods and management strategies for suspected CVT cases. Key topics include the evidence supporting anticoagulation therapy, the role of endovascular treatments, and considerations for craniectomy. Additionally, an algorithm is provided to optimize the management of CVT patients, particularly those with progressive neurological deterioration or thrombus propagation despite maximum medical therapy.

Keywords: CVT, MRI, AHA/ASA.

■ INTRODUCTION

Cerebral venous thrombosis (CVT) is a rare cause of stroke due to thrombosis of intracranial venous sinuses and veins and characterized by a wide range of clinical presentations, predisposing factors, and variable clinical outcomes. Accurate and timely diagnosis of CVT is essential, as prompt and appropriate treatment significantly lowers the risk of acute complications and long-term sequelae.[1]

■ EPIDEMIOLOGY AND INDIAN PERSPECTIVES

Among stroke patients, CVT accounts for only 0.5–3% of cases in the world.[2,3] Registry-based and cohort studies indicate that CVT primarily affects individuals under 55 years of age, with two-thirds of cases occurring in women. However, this trend seems to be changing with a decrease in the postpartum CVT cases in the recent years.[4] The frequency of puerperal CVT is higher in India compared to Western countries.[5] A relatively higher incidence in the developing countries compared to the developed ones may be attributed to genetic susceptibility combined with environmental factors such as dehydration, infection, trauma and climatic influences.[5,6]

CLINICAL PRESENTATIONS

The clinical presentations of CVT vary widely and are influenced by factors such as the patient's age, the time between onset and hospitalization, the location of the thrombosis, and its extent. Common signs and symptoms of CVT include headache, focal neurologic deficits, seizures, and diffuse encephalopathy, while rarer symptoms include cavernous sinus syndrome and coma **(Table 1)**.[3,7-11]

PREDISPOSING FACTORS

A number of predisposing factors have been identified to contribute to CVT which can be classified into transient and chronic. Among the transient risk factors, pregnancy, postpartum, oral contraceptives (54–71%), and hormone replacement therapy (4%) constitute important factors predisposing to CVT.[9,10] Other transient factors include head and neck infections (8–11%), dehydration (2–19%), anemia, sepsis, respiratory infections, and COVID-19 (7.6%) and medications like corticosteroids, L-asparaginase, thalidomide, and tamoxifen. Among the chronic factors, obesity (23%), thyroid disease, nephrotic syndrome, and inflammatory bowel disease (1–2%) have been identified. Malignancies such as myeloproliferative disorders (2–3%) and other types (7%) also contribute to the risk. Autoimmune conditions

TABLE 1: Clinical presentation based on location of sinus thrombosis.

Location of thrombosis	Incidence (%)	Clinical presentation
Transverse sinus	44–73%	• Asymptomatic or headaches if isolated without infarction; seizures, contralateral pyramidal symptoms • Left transverse sinus with venous infarction and vein of Labbé occlusion can cause aphasia. Extension into contiguous sinuses can lead to intracranial hypertension, consciousness disturbances, focal cerebral signs, and cranial nerve palsies (IX-XII) • Extension into cerebellar veins may cause headaches, vomiting, and limb or gait ataxia
Superior sagittal sinus	39–62%	Common symptoms include headache, blurred vision, visual loss, nausea, vomiting, cranial nerve palsy, aphasia, hemianopia, hemisensory loss, hemiparesis, and seizures. Isolated intracranial hypertension, focal symptoms from venous infarction, rarely isolated psychiatric symptoms
Sigmoid sinus	40–47%	Mastoid region pain, VI, VII, and VIII cranial nerve palsies
Deep venous system	10%	Altered sensorium, reduced arousal, diffuse encephalopathy or coma, bilateral or fluctuating alternating paresis
Cortical vein	3.7–17.1%	Focal neurological signs, seizures
Cavernous sinus	1.3–1.7%	Headache, ocular pain, chemosis, proptosis, ocular nerve palsy (III, IV, VI, and the ophthalmic division of V), and fever when infection is present

like antiphospholipid antibody (APLA) syndrome (6–17%), connective tissue diseases (systemic lupus erythematosus, Behçet disease, and sarcoidosis; 1%), and other genetic thrombophilias (31–41%) such as prothrombin 20210A mutation, factor V Leiden mutation, *MTHFR* (C677T) polymorphism, and antithrombin deficiency, JAK2, protein C or protein S deficiency (which can be genetic or acquired) are significant factors. Mechanical factors include head trauma (1–3%), neurosurgical procedures, jugular vein catheterizations (1–2% iatrogenic), compressive lesions of venous sinuses such as meningioma, dural arteriovenous fistula, and COVID-19 vaccine induced.[2] The importance of predisposing factor is treatment of underlying condition and duration of anticoagulation.

■ INVESTIGATIONS

Neuroimaging

The noncontrast CT scan of the head serves as an initial diagnostic tool, commonly used in hospitals for suspected stroke or acute headache cases. In approximately one-third of patients, specific signs such as hyperdensity in the venous sinus or deep veins can be observed, sometimes referred to as the dense triangle sign (indicating high attenuation in the sagittal sinus or deep cerebral veins in a triangular shape) or the cord sign (indicating high attenuation due to thrombus in the transverse sinus). The cashew nut sign— seen with isolated cortical vein thrombosis on CT is a hemorrhagic lesion with shape of cashew nut. Additionally, CT scans can reveal ischemic areas that do not conform to arterial boundaries, often accompanied by some degree of hemorrhagic transformation, as well as parenchymal or subarachnoid hemorrhages, and signs of edema. However, CT scans may appear normal in up to 30% of patients and, when abnormal, lack specificity. Therefore, all patients suspected of CVT require further imaging beyond a noncontrast CT scan.[2]

According to the European Stroke Organisation (ESO) guidelines, confirmation of the diagnosis typically involves MR venography or CT venography. CT venography due to its method of visualizing the lumen rather than flow offers excellent diagnostic accuracy (sensitivity of 95% and specificity of 91%) compared to the gold standard of digital subtraction angiography (DSA). CT venography can depict absent flow in thrombosed veins or sinuses and partial circumferential enhancement of thrombosed venous sinuses, such as the empty delta sign. However, false positives may occur due to normal sinus hypoplasia or arachnoid granulations. MR venography, utilizing time-of-flight sequences, also allows assessment of absent flow in thrombosed sinuses without the need for contrast medium, albeit with a higher risk of false positives, particularly in cases of nondominant (hypoplastic) transverse sinus.[2,3]

Magnetic resonance imaging stands out as the most sensitive modality for detecting thrombus material, utilizing sequences sensitive to the magnetic susceptibility effects of paramagnetic iron-containing blood components, such as T2*-weighted gradient echo or susceptibility-weighted imaging (SWI). The appearance of the clot on various MRI sequences varies depending on its age, which aids in estimating the likely onset of CVT. MRI also excels in fully assessing parenchymal involvement, encompassing ischemia, hemorrhages, edema, and swelling. Additionally, thrombosed sinuses appearing hyperintense on diffusion-weighted imaging are reported to have a reduced recanalization rate.[2,3]

Catheter intra-arterial DSA should be reserved for confirming the diagnosis only when CT venography or MR venography results are inconclusive or when there is suspicion of a dural arteriovenous fistula. The relationship between dural arteriovenous fistulas and CVT remains complex and not fully elucidated. In rare instances, a dural arteriovenous fistula can complicate CVT, potentially due to arteriovenous pathways opening in the sinus wall during occlusion or recanalization. Early detection of these fistulas using intra-arterial DSA is crucial for timely intervention, such as embolization. Conversely, CVT can occur concurrently with the development of an arteriovenous fistula. Regardless of the temporal relationship, clinicians must recognize the possibility of these pathologies coexisting and understand their specific treatment requirements. Isolated cortical vein thrombosis is typically well visualized on susceptibility-weighted sequences but may occasionally necessitate confirmation via intra-arterial DSA due to diagnostic challenges.[2,3]

Based on 2011 American Heart Association (AHA) recommendations, for patients with idiopathic intracranial hypertension symptoms, imaging of the cerebral venous system is recommended to exclude CVT (Class I; Level of Evidence C). In patients with lobar intracerebral hemorrhage of unknown cause or cerebral infarction that extends beyond typical arterial boundaries, imaging of the cerebral venous system is recommended (Class I; Level of Evidence C). Additionally, for those with headaches featuring atypical characteristics, imaging is reasonable to rule out CVT (Class IIa; Level of Evidence C).[3]

As per AHA 2024 guidelines, all patients suspected of having CVT, routine blood tests, including a complete blood count, biochemistry panel, prothrombin time, and activated partial thromboplastin time, should be done (Class I; Level of Evidence C). Additionally, screening for potential prothrombotic conditions like contraceptive use, underlying inflammatory disease, or infections is recommended during the initial assessment, with specific guidelines for thrombophilia testing detailed in the long-term management section (Class I; Level of Evidence C). D-dimer measurement, a fibrin degradation product, helps exclude DVT or pulmonary embolism when combined with pretest probability assessment. Although some small, methodologically limited studies showed high sensitivity for identifying CVT, this was not universally confirmed. Hence, in the presence of a strong clinical possibility of CVT, a normal D-dimer level does not preclude further evaluation. With regards to cerebrospinal fluid (CSF) analysis, unless meningitis is suspected, this is not typically useful in CVT cases with or without focal neurological abnormalities and radiographic confirmation. Elevated opening pressure, cell counts, and protein levels, though common in CVT, their absence does not rule out CVT.[3,8]

Risk Factor Analysis Including Genetic Testing

Routine thrombophilia screening aimed at reducing the risk of death or disability in CVT patients is not recommended. However, thrombophilia screening may be considered for patients with a high pre-test probability of severe thrombophilia, such as those with a personal or family history of venous thrombosis, young age at CVT onset, or CVT occurring without a transient or permanent risk factor, to prevent recurrent venous thrombotic events. Hence, testing for protein C, protein S, antithrombin deficiency, antiphospholipid syndrome, prothrombin *G20210A* mutation, factor V Leiden, and *MTHFR* gene mutation may be beneficial for managing CVT patients. Protein C, protein S, and antithrombin deficiency is typically done 2–4 weeks after anticoagulation ends, as it has limited value during the acute phase or in patients on warfarin (Class IIa; Level of Evidence B). A two-stage genome-wide case–control study has identified a locus associated with an increased risk of CVT.[3,11,12]

MANAGEMENT

The therapeutic management options that are commonly used in the management of CVT include unfractionated heparin (UFH), low-molecular weight heparin (LMWH), vitamin K antagonist (VKA), and direct oral anticoagulants (DOACs) **(Table 2)**.

- *Anticoagulation*: The goals of anticoagulation therapy in CVT are to prevent thrombus growth, promote recanalization, and prevent recurrent venous thromboembolism (VTE) events. The AHA/American Stroke Association and European management guidelines for CVT recommend initially using LMWH over UFH, followed by oral VKAs for 3–12 months in cases of transient risk factors, or indefinitely for chronic major risk factors for thrombosis or recurrent VTE. LMWH is preferred in the acute treatment of CVT due to its practical administration, more predictable anticoagulation effects, lower risk of thrombocytopenia,

TABLE 2: Recent clinical trials on anticoagulation in CVT.

Trial name	Drug used	Sample size	Methods	Results
RE-SPECT CVT	Dabigatran vs. Warfarin	120	International prospective trial. Randomized 1:1 to warfarin (target INR 2.0–3.0) or dabigatran 150 mg twice daily for 6 months after 5–15 days of lead-in parenteral anticoagulation. Excluded individuals with malignancy, CNS infection, trauma, and pregnancy	No recurrent VTEs in either group. Major hemorrhages: 1 GI bleeding (dabigatran group), 2 intracerebral hemorrhages (warfarin group)
SECRET	Rivaroxaban vs. Warfarin/LMWH	53	Phase II trial. Randomized 1:1 to rivaroxaban 20 mg daily or standard-of-care anticoagulation (Warfarin target INR 2.0–3.0 or LMWH) for at least 6 months. Excluded individuals with pregnancy and antiphospholipid antibody syndrome	No safety concerns with early DOAC initiation. Rivaroxaban group had 1 recurrent CVT, 1 symptomatic ICH, and 2 clinically relevant nonmajor bleeding events. No VTE recurrence or bleeding events in the control group
ACTION-CVT	Various DOACs (Apixaban/Rivaroxaban/Dabigatran vs. VKA)	845	Large retrospective international study. Compared VKA with DOACs (apixaban 67%, rivaroxaban 18%, dabigatran 14%, multiple DOACs 3%). Excluded individuals with malignancy, antiphospholipid antibody syndrome, and pregnancy	No significant difference in recurrent VTE rates. DOAC group had a reduced risk of major hemorrhage, primarily intracerebral hemorrhage. No differences in recanalization rates between groups

(CVT: cerebral venous thrombosis; DOAC: directly acting oral anticoagulants; ICH: intracranial hemorrhage; INR: international normalized ratio; LMWH: low-molecular weight heparin; VKA: vitamin K antagonist; VTE: venous thromboembolism) and trends toward better outcomes in meta-analyses, although these trends do not reach statistical significance. The presence of venous hemorrhage is not a contraindication for anticoagulation. Whether the degree of venous recanalization should determine the duration of anticoagulation remains uncertain.[2,3]

- *Direct oral anticoagulation*: There has been recent emergence of evidence on the role of DOACs in CVT. RE-SPECT CVT was an international trial comparing dabigatran to Warfarin in 120 CVT patients, randomized 1:1. Participants received either dabigatran 150 mg twice daily or warfarin with a target INR of 2.0–3.0 for 6 months, following 5–15 days of parenteral anticoagulation. The trial excluded those with malignancy, central nervous system (CNS) infection, trauma, or pregnancy. Both groups had no recurrent VTE, with one major hemorrhage (1.7%) in the dabigatran group and two (3.3%) in the warfarin group. SECRET, a phase II trial, randomized 53 CVT patients to rivaroxaban 20 mg daily or standard anticoagulation for 6 months, without lead-in parenteral anticoagulation. Exclusions included pregnancy and antiphospholipid syndrome. The rivaroxaban group had one recurrent CVT (3.8%), one symptomatic intracerebral hemorrhage (3.8%), and two nonmajor bleeding events (7.7%). No VTE recurrence or bleeding occurred in the control group. ACTION-CVT, a retrospective study of 845 CVT patients on VKA or DOACs (apixaban 67%, rivaroxaban 18%, and dabigatran 14%), found no difference in recurrent VTE rates (adjusted hazard ratio 0.94) but noted a reduced risk of major hemorrhage with DOACs (adjusted hazard ratio 0.35), primarily due to lower intracerebral hemorrhage risk. Recanalization rates were similar. A systematic review of three trials and 16 studies found similar rates of recurrent VTE, major hemorrhage, and recanalization with DOACs and VKAs (42.9% vs. 42.3%; relative risk 0.98). Current evidence supports transitioning to DOACs or VKAs after a period of parenteral anticoagulation, but optimal duration (5–15 days vs. shorter periods) of parental anticoagulation remains uncertain.[2]

In patients with APLA syndrome, DOACs have shown higher risks of recurrent thromboembolic events compared to warfarin. However, for cancer patients, DOACs have demonstrated noninferiority to LMWH in preventing VTE. The role of antiplatelet agents after stopping oral anticoagulation in CVT remains uncertain, with limited evidence available. Studies focusing on secondary prevention of VTE have indicated that aspirin is more effective than placebo [hazard ratio 0.68 (95% confidence interval (CI) 0.51–0.90); $p = 0.008$]. Given that CVT patients are typically younger and may have longer exposure to aspirin over their lifetimes, the potential benefits should be weighed carefully against individual patient characteristics in shared decision-making **(Tables 2 and 3; Fig. 1)**.[2]

Management of Late Complications

- *Headache:* During follow-up, about 50% of CVT patients experience headaches, which are usually primary and unrelated to CVT. Studies show a mix of residual headaches, migraines, and tension-type headaches. Severe headaches requiring bed rest or hospital admission occurred in 11–14% of patients. Persistent or severe headaches should be investigated to rule out recurrent CVT and secondary dural AV fistula.[3]
- *Seizures*: Post-CVT seizures, either focal or generalized, affect 5–32% of patients, mostly within the 1st year. Risk

TABLE 3: Management options of anticoagulants in cerebral venous thrombosis patients.

	UFH	LMWH	VKA	DOAC
AHA/ASA guidelines	Recommended, IIa, LoE: B	Recommended, IIa, LoE: B	Recommended, IIb, LoE: C	NA
ESO guidelines	Recommended (moderate, strong)	Recommended (low, weak)	Recommended (very low, weak)	Not recommended (very low, weak)
Dose	1,000 IU/h	Enoxaparin 60 mg SC Q12H	2–5 mg OD	• Rivaroxaban 20 mg QD • Apixaban 5 mg BD • Dabigatran 150 mg BD
Therapy duration	Acute stage until no indication for surgical or EVT	Acute stage until no indication for surgical or EVT	3–6 months in transient cases	3–6 months in transient cases
Monitoring	aPTT 1.5–2.5 times the control	Nil	Target INR 2–3	NA
Remarks	HITT to consider in case of thrombocytopenia	Avoid in renal failure	• Reduces protein C and S, hence, requires bridging therapy • Avoid in pregnancy	• Avoid in pregnancy • Sudden discontinuation an lead to thrombosis

(DOAC: direct oral anticoagulant; LMWH: low-molecular weight heparin; UFH: unfractionated heparin; VKA: vitamin K antagonist)

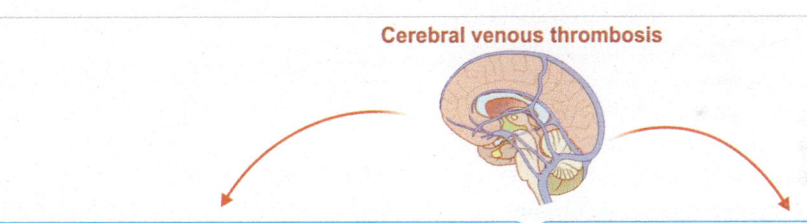

Cerebral venous thrombosis

Evaluation for risk factors and etiologies:
- Clinical evaluation for malignancy, neuroinfection, dehydration, otitis, mastoiditis, rheumatological disorders
- CBC, hematocrit
- Renal and liver function tests
- PT/APTT/INR

Additional tests when indicated:
- Pregnancy testing
- *Inflammatory panel:* Antiphospholipid antibody panel, c-ANCA, p-ANCA, ANA, HLA-B51
- *Thrombophilia panel:* Protein C, S, ATIII, homocysteine levels; Factor V, MTHFR, JAK-2, V617F prothrombin gene mutations, MTHFR
- *Hematologic panel:* Iron studies, CD55, 59, Hb electrophoresis, anti-platelet factor 1 and 2
- *Infective panel:* HIV, COVID-19, sepsis

Management:
- LMWH>UFH *(ICH due to CVT is not contra indication)*
- *Severe CVT:* Decompressive surgery
- *Role of EVT:* Need for further studies
- *Transition to OAC:* DOACs or warfarin
- *Transient:* 3 to 12 months
- Recurrent VTE/High-risk
- *Thrombophilia:* Indefinite
- **Pregnancy:* LMWH
- *Imaging shows thrombus propagation with clinical progression:* EVT or intrasinus thrombolysis

* Choice of anticoagulation

FIG. 1: Management of cerebral venous sinus thrombosis.

(APTT: activated partial thromboplastin time; CVT: cerebral venous thrombosis; DOAC: direct oral anticoagulant; ICH: intracranial hemorrhage; INR: international normalized ratio; LMWH: low-molecular weight heparin; PT: prothrombin time; UFH: unfractionated heparin; VTE: venous thromboembolism)

factors include hemorrhagic lesions, early seizures, and paresis. Post-CVT epilepsy occurs in about 5% of patients. Antiepileptic drugs are recommended for those with parenchymal lesions who present with a single seizure. However, it remains unclear whether to initiate treatment in patients who have experienced a seizure but lack supratentorial brain lesions, or in those with lesions but no clinical seizures.

When administering antiepileptic drugs, it is crucial to select medications that do not interfere with planned anticoagulant therapies. Currently, there is no established consensus on the optimal duration of treatment for seizures associated with CVT. Based on existing data, treatment is usually advised for at least 1 year in cases involving seizures linked to edema, infarction, or hemorrhage.[13]

- *Visual loss*: Severe visual loss from CVT is rare (2-4%) but can result from prolonged papilledema leading to optic atrophy and blindness. Patients with visual complaints should undergo a comprehensive neuro-ophthalmological evaluation. There is no specific regimen for managing impending vision loss in CVT. Although there are no randomized trials on prolonged use of mannitol and glycerol for antiedema, some observational studies suggest their use with daily monitoring of headaches and vision. Steroids, such as IV methylprednisolone, are generally ineffective unless vision loss is due to an autoimmune or inflammatory condition. Data on endovascular therapy and decompressive craniectomy for vision loss without parenchymal involvement are limited. Surgery may be considered for progressive vision loss despite optimal medical therapy. Few observational studies suggest that optic nerve sheath fenestration (ONSF) can be beneficial if performed correctly, and a systematic review found improvement in cases who underwent ventriculoperitoneal shunting for CVT-related vision loss.[3]
- *Dural arteriovenous fistula*: Thrombosis of the cavernous, lateral, or sagittal sinus can induce a dural arteriovenous fistula. Its exact frequency is unknown due to a lack of long-term angiographic studies, but it is low (1-3%) in cohorts without systematic follow-up. A cerebral angiogram can help identify its presence.[3]

Anticoagulation in Special Conditions

- *Cerebral venous thrombosis in neonates and children*: CVT is more common in neonates (6.4/100,000) than in children and adolescents. Early diagnosis is key in cases of headache, seizures, focal neurological deficits, coma, and situations like sepsis (including mastoiditis, Lemierre syndrome, COVID-19, and meningitis), head trauma, hypoxia, and dehydration, especially in children with preexisting conditions (congenital heart disease, cancer, anemia, and inflammatory diseases). Blood investigations comprise evaluation for platelet factor 4 mutations in presence of thrombocytopenia, or JAK2 mutations in presence of high platelets and high hemoglobin. Other relevant blood work-ups comprise iron studies with or without anemia. Treatment typically involves LMWH or UFH, with more invasive procedures considered for severe cases. While anticoagulation in neonates is debated, it is generally recommended due to the risk of thrombus propagation. CVT in children has a 3% mortality rate and a 6% recurrence rate, often due to lack of anticoagulation and recanalization. Recent trials, such as Kids-DOTT and EINSTEIN-Jr, have explored the duration and efficacy of anticoagulation, showing promising results for shorter treatment durations and the use of rivaroxaban. Despite treatment, long-term complications like epilepsy, cognitive impairment, and intracranial hypertension may occur in about 25% of cases.[3]

The Kids-DOTT trial (Multicenter Evaluation of the Duration of Therapy for Thrombosis in Children) compared 6 weeks with 3 months of anticoagulation for provoked VTE in individuals aged 4 months to 20.9 years (including 59 out of 417 patients, or 25%, with CVT). 6 weeks of anticoagulation was found to be noninferior for recurrent VTE and bleeding events. In the EINSTEIN-Jr trial (Oral Rivaroxaban in Children With Venous Thrombosis), after initial heparinization, 114 children with confirmed CVT were randomized (2:1) to 3 months of rivaroxaban or standard anticoagulation (continuing heparin or switching to oral VKAs). The primary efficacy outcome was symptomatic recurrent VTE, and the principal safety outcome was major or clinically relevant nonmajor bleeding. With 100% follow-up, none of the 73 children treated with rivaroxaban, compared to 1 of the 41 children treated with standard anticoagulation, had symptomatic recurrent VTE [absolute difference, 2.4% (95% CI −2.6 to 13.5%)]. Five patients on rivaroxaban experienced nonmajor and noncerebral bleeding, while one patient on standard anticoagulation had a major subdural bleed. Complete or partial recanalization occurred in 18 (25%) and 39 (53%) patients on rivaroxaban, and 6 (15%) and 24 (59%) patients on standard anticoagulation. No children died by the end of the 3-month study treatment period. Focal neurological deficits were observed in 5 (6.8%) children in the rivaroxaban group and 3 (7.3%) in the standard anticoagulation group at the study's conclusion. However, other long-term studies suggest that despite treatment, 1 in 4 children may develop late epilepsy, infantile spasms after neonatal CVT, cognitive impairment, or intracranial hypertension.[2]

- *Pregnancy and puerperium*: Pregnancy induces changes in the coagulation system that persist into the puerperium, creating a hypercoagulable state and increasing the risk of CVT. Incidence during pregnancy and puerperium ranges from 1 in 2,500 to 1 in 10,000 deliveries in Western countries, with ORs from 1.3 to 13.0. The highest risk periods are the third trimester and the first six postpartum weeks, with about 80% of pregnancy-related CVT cases occurring after delivery. Cesarean section is associated with a higher risk after adjusting for age, vascular risk factors, infections, hospital type, and location. Studies suggest the prognosis for women with pregnancy-related CVT is as good as or better than for CVT in general. VKAs, including warfarin, are contraindicated in pregnancy due to risks of fetal embryopathy and bleeding. Anticoagulation during pregnancy and early puerperium usually involves LMWH. Evidence on endovascular therapies is limited, and thrombolysis and thrombectomy are reserved for cases with neurological deterioration or thrombus propagation despite medical therapy.[14]

A systematic review of 17 studies involving 393 pregnancies found a recurrence rate of 8 per 1,000 pregnancies (95% CI 3-22), and a rate of noncerebral VTEs of 22 per 1,000 pregnancies (95% CI 11-43). There was a trend toward a lower recurrence rate in women who used antithrombotic prophylaxis. Current evidence indicates that CVT is not a contraindication for future pregnancies. Given the added risk of pregnancy for women with a history of CVT, prophylaxis with LMWH during future pregnancies and the postpartum period is likely beneficial.

- *Cerebral venous thrombosis with coexisting abnormal uterine bleeding (AUB)*: The International Society on Thrombosis and Hemostasis recommends against discontinuation of estrogen-containing contraceptives in certain patients with a strong clinical indication while they are undergoing anticoagulant treatment. The anticoagulant therapy may mitigate the prothrombotic effects of the estrogen-containing contraceptives when both are used together. An alternative form of contraception should be sought before stopping the anticoagulant therapy.[3]
- *Vaccine-induced immune thrombotic thrombocytopenia (VITT), COVID-19, and CVT:* In 2021, reports from Europe and the US reported cases of thrombocytopenia and CVT following vaccination with the AstraZeneca (ChAdOx1nCoV-19) and Janssen (Ad26.COV2.S) adenovirus-based COVID-19 vaccines. Affected patients, mostly women aged 18–77, developed symptoms 5–24 days after vaccination, with headache being the most common symptom. All patients had thrombocytopenia, and in the UK, 23 patients had antibodies to platelet factor 4. It is believed that DNA from adenovirus-infected cells bonded to platelet factor 4, triggering autoantibody production. Although rare, CVT in VITT has a poor prognosis, with initial studies showing mortality rates of 39–61%. A global study found 26 VITT cases among 2,313 CVT admissions over 2 years, resulting in 6 deaths, with COVID-19 infection present in 7.6% of CVT admissions.

Pharmacovigilance data indicated a lower incidence of CVT after mRNA vaccines (1–5/10,000 for BNT162b2 and mRNA-1273) compared to adenovirus-based vaccines (13/10,000 for ChAdOx1 nCoV-19), with no evidence of VITT after mRNA vaccines. For suspected VITT, testing for platelet factor 4 antibodies is recommended. Treatment includes avoiding heparin products, administering intravenous immunoglobulin and steroids, and using nonheparin anticoagulants like argatroban or fondaparinux, transitioning to DOACs once platelet count recovers.[2]

Reperfusion Therapies

Theoretical advantages of endovascular treatment (EVT) for CVT include potentially quicker recanalization, but its impact on improving outcomes over medical therapy, especially in unselected patient populations, remains uncertain. Over the past decade, various studies have explored mechanical thrombectomy (including balloon-assisted or aspiration/vacuum systems), intrasinus thrombolysis, combinations of thrombectomy and thrombolysis, intra-arterial thrombolysis, and intrasinus stenting, yielding controversial findings regarding safety and complication rates. The multicenter randomized TO-ACT trial (Thrombolysis or Anticoagulation for CVT) indicated no clinical benefit from EVT compared to standard anticoagulation therapy in patients with severe CVT. Larger studies and meta-analyses have similarly found EVT associated with higher mortality rates and no demonstrable clinical benefit.[2]

Currently, EVT serves as a salvage therapy for patients experiencing clinical deterioration, treatment failure, or those with contraindications to standard therapies. In a systematic review encompassing 10 studies with 339 CVT patients treated with EVT, authors reported complete or partial postoperative recanalization in 90.0% of cases, rising to 95.2% during follow-up. The complication rate was 10.3%. Additionally, balloon-assisted MT is safe and cost-effective in developing countries like India.[15] There is insufficient current evidence to determine the superiority of any specific EVT technique (such as stent retrievers, microcatheters, aspiration catheters, or aspiration pump systems) over other therapeutic approaches.[16-20]

Management of Raised Intracranial Pressure and Decompression Craniectomy

Management of elevated intracranial pressure during the acute phase of CVT, attributed to conditions like space-occupying brain edema, infarction, or intracranial hemorrhage, is critical to prevent severe brain injury and potential mortality. Patients at risk or presenting with elevated intracranial pressure should ideally be treated in a neurological critical care unit with immediate access to endovascular and neurosurgical teams. Medical interventions include osmotic therapy (e.g., mannitol), controlled hyperventilation (targeting PCO_2 levels of 30–35 mm Hg), and positioning the patient with elevated head of bed. The efficacy of therapeutic lumbar puncture in acute CVT is uncertain. Moreover, it is contraindicated in patients with significant brain lesions at risk of herniation.[2]

Carbonic anhydrase inhibitors like acetazolamide lack supporting evidence in CVT but may benefit patients with severe headaches or visual threats. Corticosteroids are not recommended unless underlying inflammatory conditions like Behçet's disease or systemic lupus erythematosus are present.[2]

- *Topiramate*: Topiramate blocks voltage-gated sodium channels, inhibits kainate-type glutamate receptors, reduces L-type voltage-sensitive calcium currents, enhances GABA-mediated chloride channel activity, inhibits carbonic anhydrase, and increases potassium conductance. Additionally, it significantly inhibits the release of calcitonin gene-related peptide in ganglion cell cultures. These mechanisms collectively reduce neuronal excitation and help in reduction of headaches.[2]

Decompression Craniectomy

In cases of brain herniation or significant midline shift (termed "malignant CVT"), medical management alone may prove inadequate. Decompressive craniectomy offers a potential life-saving intervention by allowing brain swelling to expand and possibly improving collateral vein drainage in CVT. It is recommended for patients experiencing acute severe CVT with parenchymal lesions and impending herniation, as it represents a critical, life-saving intervention. Factors contributing to poorer outcomes include age over 50 years, midline shift exceeding 10 mm, and complete obliteration of basal cisterns. A sustained intracranial pressure exceeding 20 cmH_2O is also suggested as a potential indication for surgical intervention. Despite these recommendations, there are no randomized controlled trials evaluating the efficacy of this surgical approach in the current literature. However, a systematic review and meta-analysis of 51 studies involving 483 CVT patients indicated that performing surgery within 48 hours of admission may reduce mortality [odds ratio (OR) 0.26 (95% CI 0.10–0.69)] and lead to improved functional outcomes.[2,11]

The optimal timing of anticoagulation following hemicraniectomy varies widely, typically initiated between 24 hours and 8 days postsurgery. Replacing the bone flap, often done after 3–6 months when brain swelling subsides, is standard practice. Given the likelihood of significant functional impairments in survivors of hemicraniectomy for CVT, thorough discussions with patients or their families are crucial before proceeding with intervention. Ventricular shunting has not demonstrated efficacy in preventing death or herniation in CVT-related intracranial hypertension and is therefore not recommended.[21]

RECANALIZATION

A recent meta-analysis examined how recanalization impacts specific outcomes in CVT. The absence of recanalization was consistently linked to worse functional outcomes, including chronic headache and recurrence of thrombosis.[22]

PROGNOSIS

Cerebral venous thrombosis typically results in a favorable outcome, with approximately 75% of patients achieving complete functional recovery; however, around 15% either die or experience dependency. In the acute phase, factors associated with poorer outcomes include male gender, advanced age, confusion or coma, intracranial hemorrhage, involvement of deep veins, infection, and malignancy. Cognitive decline is often overlooked, particularly in cases involving deep vein thrombosis, affecting up to one-third of patients. The risk of recurrent CVT is relatively low, estimated at 2-7%, and slightly higher for systemic thromboembolism (4-7%). Patients with severe thrombophilic disorders or those who discontinue anticoagulant therapy prematurely are identified as being at highest risk for recurrence.[2]

CONCLUSION

Cerebral venous thrombosis requires high suspicion in patients presenting with common symptoms and known predisposing conditions such as pregnancy, puerperium, oral contraceptive use, thrombophilia, or in young women. New predisposing factors identified since the last report include obesity, COVID-19, and vaccine-induced thrombocytopenia. MRI/MRV is the preferred noninvasive method for diagnosing CVT, though CT/CTV can be used in centers with limited resources or when pretest probability is low. For diagnosing cortical venous thrombosis, contrast-enhanced MRV, gradient-recalled echo, or SWI is recommended. Initial treatment typically involves parenteral heparin followed by oral VKAs for 3-12 months, or indefinitely for those with thrombophilia or recurrent VTE. DOACs are also a safe and effective alternative to VKAs. The use of venous recanalization seen on subsequent CTV or MRV to determine the duration of anticoagulation is still uncertain.

In the absence of RCTs, endovascular therapies can be considered when there is evidence of thrombus propagation, neurological deterioration despite best medical therapy, or for those with contraindications to anticoagulation. Decompressive surgery, despite limited evidence, can be life-saving and improve outcomes in cases with brain herniation. Pregnant women with CVT should continue full-dose LMWH throughout pregnancy and switch to LMWH or VKAs with an INR target of 2.0-3.0 for at least 6 weeks postpartum. Future pregnancies are generally safe for women with a history of CVT, with recommended LMWH prophylaxis during pregnancy and postpartum. CVT is more common in neonates, often linked to infections or anemia. The recommended treatment includes parenteral anticoagulation as the initial treatment followed by LMWH, VKAs, or rivaroxaban for at least 6 weeks.[2,23]

REFERENCES

1. Jan S. Thrombosis of the Cerebral Veins and Sinuses. N Engl J Med. 2005;352(17):1791-8.
2. Saposnik G, Bushnell C, Coutinho JM, Field TS, Furie KL, Galadanci N, et al. Diagnosis and Management of Cerebral Venous Thrombosis: A Scientific Statement from the American Heart Association. Stroke. 2024;55(3):e77-e90.
3. Saposnik G, Barinagarrementeria F, Brown RD, Bushnell CD, Cucchiara B, Cushman M, et al. Diagnosis and Management of Cerebral Venous Thrombosis: a statement for healthcare professionals from the American Heart Association/American Stroke Association. Stroke. 2011;42:1158-92.
4. Miraclin AT, Prasad JD, Ninan GA, Gowri M, Bal D, Shaikh AIA, et al. Cerebral venous sinus thrombosis: changing trends in the incidence, age and gender (findings from the CMC Vellore CVT registry). Stroke Vasc Neurol. 2024;9(3):252-7.
5. Dash D, Prasad K, Joseph L. Cerebral venous thrombosis: An Indian perspective. Neurol India. 2015;63(3):318-28.
6. Aaron S, Lakshmanan J, Sudarsanam TD, Benjamin K, Durairaj J, Mathew V, et al. Cerebral venous thrombosis, seasonal trends, and climatic influence: A region-specific study. Ann Indian Acad Neurol. 2020;23:522-7.
7. Kalita J, Singh V, Misra U. A study of hyperhomocysteinemia in cerebral venous sinus thrombosis. Indian J Med Res. 2020;152:584-94.
8. Kulkarni GB, Mustare V, Abbas MM. Profile of patients with cerebral venous sinus thrombosis with cerebellar involvement. J Stroke Cerebrovasc Dis. 2014;23:1106-11.
9. Ulivi L, Squitieri M, Cohen H, Cowley P, Werring DJ. Cerebral venous thrombosis: A practical guide. Pract Neurol. 2020;20(5):356-67.
10. Field TS, Hill MD. Cerebral Venous Thrombosis: We Should Ask the Right Questions to Get Better Answers. Stroke. 2019;50(6):1598-604.
11. Borhani-Haghighi A, Hooshmandi E. Cerebral venous thrombosis: a practical review. Postgrad Med J. 2024;100(1180):68-83.
12. Cotlarciuc I, Marjot T, Khan MS, Hiltunen S, Haapaniemi E, Metso TM, et al. Towards the genetic basis of cerebral venous thrombosis-the BEAST Consortium: a study protocol on behalf of the ISGC (International Stroke Genetics Consortium) and BEAST investigators. BMJ Open. 2016;6(11):e012351.
13. Miranda B, Aaron S, Arauz A, Barinagarrementeria F, Borhani-Haghighi A, Carvalho M, et al. The benefit of EXtending oral antiCOAgulation treatment (EXCOA) after acute cerebral vein thrombosis (CVT): EXCOA-CVT cluster randomized trial protocol. Int J Stroke. 2018;13:771-4.
14. Durmuş B, Yperzeele L, Zuurbier SM. Cerebral venous thrombosis in women of childbearing age: diagnosis, treatment, and prophylaxis during a future pregnancy. Ther Adv Neurol Disord. 2020;13:1756286420945169.
15. Alwan A, Miraclin AT, Bal D, Moses V, Mannam P, Ahmed M, et al. Management of Severe Cerebral Venous Sinus Thrombosis Using Mechanical Balloon Assisted Thrombectomy. Stroke: Vasc Interv Neurol. 2023;3(1):1-5.
16. Palanisamy P, Kramadhari H, Badachi S, Kumar GGS, Aggipothu B, Mathew T, et al. Endovascular management of cerebral venous thrombosis: a tertiary-centre experience. Pol J Radiol. 2023;88:e349-55.
17. Piano M, Romi A, Cervo A, Gatti A, Macera A, Pero G, et al. Endovascular Treatment of Cerebral Vein Thrombosis: Safety and Effectiveness in the Thrombectomy Era. Diagnostics (Basel). 2023;13(13):2248.
18. Lee SK, Mokin M, Hetts SW, Fifi JT, Bousser MG, Fraser JF. Current endovascular strategies for cerebral venous thrombosis: Report of the SNIS Standards and Guidelines Committee. J Neurointerv Surg. 2018;10:803-10.
19. Nepal G, Kharel S, Bhagat R, Coghlan MA, Yadav JK, Goeschl S, et al. Safety and efficacy of endovascular thrombectomy in patients with severe cerebral venous thrombosis: A meta-analysis. J Cent Nerv Syst Dis. 2022;14:11795735221131736.
20. Coutinho JM, Zuurbier SM, Bousser MG, Ji X, Canhão P, Roos YB, et al. Effect of endovascular treatment with medical management vs standard care on severe cerebral venous thrombosis: The TO-ACT randomized clinical trial. JAMA Neurol. 2020;77:966-73.
21. Siddiqui FM, Dandapat S, Banerjee C, Zuurbier SM, Johnson M, Stam J, et al. Mechanical Thrombectomy in Cerebral Venous Thrombosis. Stroke. 2015;46(5):1263-8.
22. Kim DJ, Honig A, Alimohammadi A, Sepehry AA, Zhou LW, Field TS. Recanalization and outcomes after cerebral venous thrombosis: a systematic review and meta-analysis. Res Pract Thromb Haemost. 2023;7(3):100143.
23. Ferro JM, Bousser MG, Canhão P, et al. European Stroke Organization guideline for the diagnosis and treatment of cerebral venous thrombosis – Endorsed by the European Academy of Neurology. Eur Stroke J. 2017;2(3):195-221.

CHAPTER 9

Misinterpretations in Vessel Wall Magnetic Resonance Imaging: Essential Insights

Pallav Bhatter, Rajsrinivas Parthasarathy, Vipul Gupta

ABSTRACT

High-resolution intracranial vessel wall magnetic resonance imaging (VW-MRI) has emerged as a critical tool for the direct visualization and characterization of vessel wall abnormalities. Applications of VW-MRI include evaluating atherosclerosis, with the ability to differentiate between positive and negative remodeling and assess plaque burden. It also plays a crucial role in identifying the location of plaques and assessing stroke risk. Additionally, VW-MRI is instrumental in diagnosing and differentiating between various nonatherosclerotic conditions such as central nervous system vasculitis, reversible cerebral vasoconstriction syndrome (RCVS), and Moyamoya disease. The technique aids in assessing aneurysm stability and recognizing high-risk features. Understanding the challenges is essential for accurate diagnosis and effective management. This article highlights critical insights into these misinterpretations, aiming to improve diagnostic precision in vessel wall MRI.

Keywords: VW-MRI, Plaques, Stroke risk, RCVS, Technique.

■ INTRODUCTION

High-resolution intracranial vessel wall magnetic resonance imaging (VW-MRI) is becoming more and more popular as a means of directly visualizing the vessel wall. While computed tomography angiography (CTA), magnetic resonance angiography (MRA), and digital subtraction angiography (DSA) techniques can identify anomalies of the vessel lumen, they may not be able to fully characterize diseases that reside within the vessel wall.

■ WHAT IS VW-MRI?

Vessel wall imaging is an MRI-based high-resolution vascular wall imaging (HR-VWI) that allows evaluation of arterial walls in the submillimeter range. VWI serves as a complementary tool to luminal wall imaging technique in disease detection and differentiation. This method can increase diagnostic specificity due to its ability to characterize changes in the vessel wall. It is also capable of identifying nonstenotic and small vessel disease, poorly defined by luminal imaging.

■ HOW INTRACRANIAL VESSELS ARE DIFFERENT TO EXTRACRANIAL VESSELS?

The artery wall consists of three main layers—the inner intima is usually very thin in healthy human arteries and consists of a layer of connective tissue. The next layer is called tunica media and contains many smooth muscle cells. The intima and tunica media are separated by a thin layer of tissue called the internal elastic lamina (IEL). Finally, adventitia surrounds the media.

Cerebral arteries have thinner tunica media and outer lamina than systemic vessels. Instead of the outer elastic lamina, there are fewer elastic fibers and the inner elastic lamina is fenestrated.[1] In contrast, extracranial arteries have several layers of outer elastic lamina and no inner elastic lamina. Additionally, tiny openings 1–3 µm in diameter are observed on the surface of the intracranial vessel wall connecting the tunica media to the cerebrospinal fluid (CSF); Zervas et al. argue that these tiny channels bring the CSF in contact with the deeper layers of the vessel wall, creating a network of outer membranes called rete vasorum.[1-3] This difference from systemic vessels means that intracranial arteries are nourished by diffusion of CSF, which reduces the nutrient demand from the outer membrane of the vessels.

Vasa vasorum are considered vessels in the host vessel wall and form a microvascular network, mainly in the aorta. Its main function is to supply oxygen and nutrients to the outer membrane and outer tunica media and to remove waste products, while the inner vascular layer is nourished by intimal diffusion of blood. Normally, vasa vasorum in the intracranial circulation are absent and appear only in disease state. These vessels include arteries, capillaries, and veins, which are responsible for feeding the vessel wall. Since the vasa vasora is usually present if there are more than 29 muscle layers in the tunica media, increased vessel wall thickness and hypoxemia of the lumen are some of the provoking factors for vasa vasorum formation. Vasa vasorum formation occurs when the wall thickness exceeds 350 microns.[4] They may also be seen in the proximal 1.5 cm of the intracranial segment. Two types of vasa vasorum are known: (1) the vasa vasorum interna (VVI) arising from the main artery, and (2) the vasa vasorum externa (VVE) arising from lateral branches.

> *Pearls*
> - Vasa vasorum are absent in intracranial circulation.
> - Only appear in disease state
> - May occasionally be seen in proximal 1.5 cm of ICA segment

■ PROTOCOL OF VESSEL WALL MAGNETIC RESONANCE IMAGING

The main technical requirements for intracranial VW-MR are: (1) high spatial resolution, (2) multidimensional 2D or 3D tomography, (3) multiple tissue weighting, and (4) signal suppression from luminal blood and CSF.

Normal arterial wall thicknesses are 0.2 mm and 0.3 mm, signal acquisition depends on the fact that wall thickness increases with disease and that the surrounding signal from luminal blood and adjacent tissues must be suppressed to obtain signal from the arterial wall.

High signal-to-noise ratios with a 2.0 × 0.4 × 0.4 mm voxel size are achieved at 3T than 1.5T, an advantage for intracranial VW-MR imaging and are often required providing a reasonable balance between spatial resolution and signal-to-noise ratio, for a 2–4 cm thick tissue slice at scan time of about 5–7 minutes.

■ SEQUENCES FOR VESSEL WALL MAGNETIC RESONANCE IMAGING

- T1 fat saturated black blood pre- and postcontrast (coronal, axial, and sagittal planes)

- T2 3D
- PDFS 3D
- 3D TOF MR angiography

PATIENT PREPARATION

The patient (or legal representative) should be explained about MRI, and MRI staff should assess for contraindications to MRI (claustrophobia, contraindicated intra-body metals, and pregnancy) or gadolinium-containing contrast agents (known allergic reaction to contrast agents, severe renal dysfunction).

CLINICAL INFORMATION

When requesting VW imaging, the actual clinical condition of the patient (neurological status, ability to remain immobile for long periods of time) should be reported in order to preliminarily assess the possibility of obtaining images of adequate diagnostic quality. The patient's treatment status is another important clinical characteristic for evaluating VW imaging. If a patient underwent an MRI study with contrast administration <12 hours before VW imaging, there may be residual contrast on subsequent precontrast VW images.

APPLICATIONS OF VESSEL WALL MRI IN VARIOUS PATHOLOGICAL CONDITIONS

Intracranial Arteriosclerotic Disease

Atherosclerosis is a complex disease involving inflammation, lipoprotein deposition, and intima growth.[5] In many atherosclerotic arteries, the intima is significantly thicker than in healthy arteries, calcification and necrosis are often observed.[6] Vessel wall MRI can be used to study the arterial wall architecture and identify the type of remodeling, high-risk plaques, and determine procedural risks.

Large Plaque Burden: Still not Visible on Luminal Imaging?

When a plaque forms in the arterial wall, the size of the artery continues to increase first with increasing plaque load, and the arterial lumen also shows compensatory expansion (active remodeling phase). After a certain plaque load, the outer diameter of the artery remains the same but the lumen narrows, eventually leading to negative remodeling. The threshold at which luminal narrowing begins is 40% for plaques in the coronary arteries, 65% in the proximal internal carotid artery (ICA), and 55% in the basilar artery. Compared with anterior circulation, posterior circulation has a greater probability of positive remodeling.

Positive and negative remodeling is determined by whether the area enclosed by the external elastic membranes (EEMs) at the lesion is larger or smaller compared to the adjacent reference (normal) segment. Vessel area (VA) is defined as the cross-sectional area limited by the EEM of the vessel while lumen area (LA) is defined as the cross-sectional area enclosed by the endothelium. Plaque burden is defined as the difference between the VA and LA divided by the VA. In positive remodeling, approximately 37% of intracranial plaques cannot be assessed by angiography. The VA at lesion site (LS) is larger than the VA of the reference site (RS) **(Fig. 1)**. The LA is relatively preserved. The remodeling ratio (RR), that is the ratio of VA at the LS to VA at the RS, is greater than 1.05. The plaque burden is large, but the lumen is not stenosed. Whereas, in negative remodeling, the VA at the LS is less than the VA at the RS **(Fig. 1)**. The lumen is significantly narrowed and the plaque burden is low. In the case of negative remodeling, the remodeling coefficient is <0.95. **Table 1** lists the differences between positive and negative remodeling.

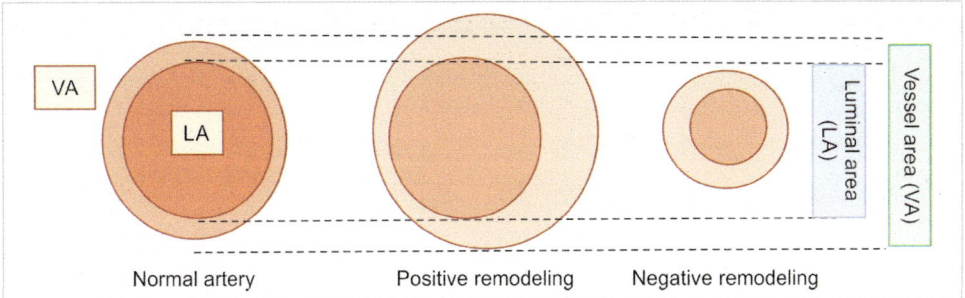

FIG. 1: Diagrammatic representation comparing the remodeling patterns in artery.

TABLE 1: Comparison between positive and negative remodeling pattern of the artery.

Positive remodeling	Negative remodeling
VA (at lesion site) > VA (at reference site)	VA (at lesion site) < VA (at reference site)
LA preserved	LA reduced
RR > 1.05	RR < 0.95

(LA: lumen area; VA: vessel area)

Does Plaque Location Determine the Stroke Risk?

Angioplasty and stenting push the plaque outward to the arterial wall and shift the plaque contents on the ostium of the perforator which can lead to plaque migration and subsequent occlusion of branch and perforating arteries. In this regard, VWI helps to map the location of the plaque and its relationship to branch and perforating arteries. In a study by Xu et al.[7] of 92 stenotic middle cerebral arteries (MCAs), plaques were more frequently found on the ventral (44.8%) and inferior (31.7%) walls compared to the superior (14.3%) and dorsal (9.0%) walls. In symptomatic MCA stenosis, plaques were more frequently found in the superior wall. In basilar artery stenosis, Huang et al.[8] studied 38 symptomatic patients and found that plaques were more frequently present in the ventral wall (21.6%) than in the dorsal (6.3%), left (4.6%), and right (2.6%) sides. Patients whose plaques are located near the ostium of the penetrating vessel are more likely to have a perforator vascular stroke after stenting because of the "snow-ploughing" effect.[7,8]

What is Threatened Morphology?

Plaque extending up to or across the ostia and causing greater than 50% ostial narrowing has an 80% chance of occlusion during the procedure **(Fig. 2)**.

> *Pearl*
>
> Risk of ostial occlusion with balloon angioplasty and stenting is close to 80% when the ostial stenosis is >50%.

What Role does Flow Dynamics Play in Plaque Formation?

At common carotid artery (CCA) bifurcation, there is a flow divider. Whenever the blood flows through the CCA into the ICA and external carotid artery (ECA), it is separated from the outer wall of the ICA. This zone is denoted as the separation zone. A dead space is formed between the flow jet and the arterial wall. The high velocity jet that hits the flow divider takes a circumferential path and reaches the dead space. By this time, the flow velocity significantly drops. This low velocity–low shear jet goes retrograde and then antegrade. The other pattern this jet takes is that of a helical one and

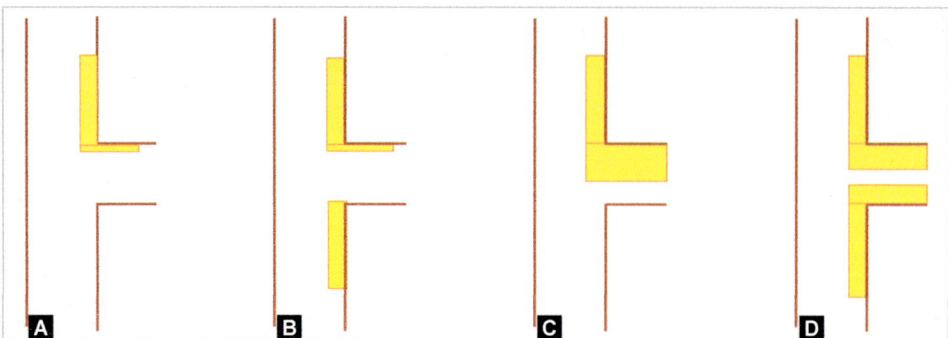

FIGS. 2A TO D: Line diagram demonstrating the morphology of threatened plaque in relation to vessel side wall. (A and B) show nonthreatened morphology while (C and D) plaques show threatened morphology.

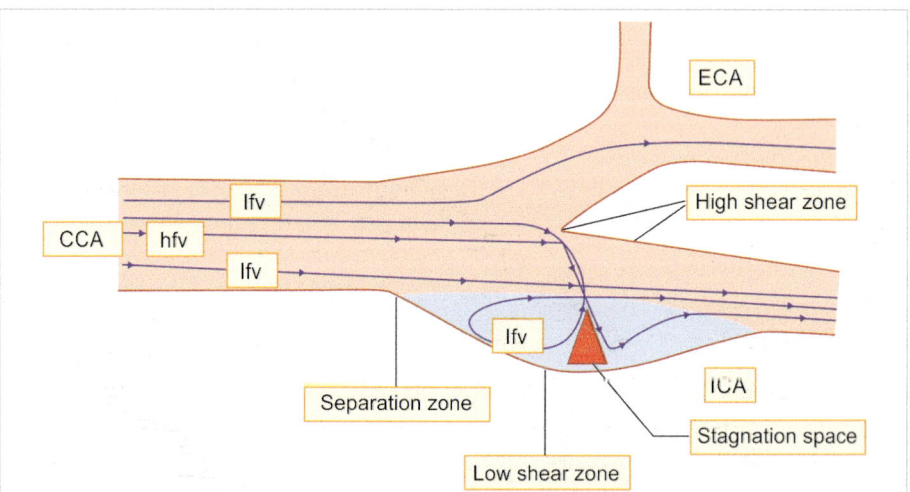

FIG. 3: Diagrammatic representation showing the mechanism of plaque formation along the carotid bifurcation. (hfv: high-flow volume; lfv: low-flow volume)

goes antegrade (as represented in **Fig. 3**). The low velocity results in low shear and this results in tumor necrosis factor (TNF) and interleukin (IL)-1β activation. These inflammatory mediators promote high-risk plaque formation and subsequently plaque rupture. Flow dynamics play a key role in determining which wall of the artery is prone for plaque formation. In certain circumstances when there are no vascular risk factors, the curvature alone may be the key contributory factor for plaque formation. Two-thirds of strokes are due to such positively remodeled plaques and the mechanism is plaque rupture. In a third of patients, high shear along the wall of the stenosis in negatively remodeled arteries causes erosion of endothelium resulting in thrombus formation and migration (no plaque rupture occurs as plaque is stable).[9]

> **Pearls: Stroke mechanism**
> - *High-flow velocity*: High shear stress—negative remodeling—erosion/dissection—stable plaque (a third)
> - *Low-flow velocity*: Low shear stress—positive remodeling—plaque rupture— unstable plaque (two-thirds)

> **Key pearls**
> - Eccentricity
> - Fibrous cap is T2 hyperintense.
> - Plaque contents are T1 and T2 hypointense.
> - Post rupture plaque enhancement lasts for 4–8 weeks.

Magnetic resonance imaging VWI features of plaque:
- Plaque contents **(Fig. 4)**
- *Fibrous cap*: T2 hyperintense
- *Lipid core*:
  - Cholesterol and cholesterol esters, not triglyceride
  - Thus hypointense on T1 and T2 WI
- *Intraplaque hemorrhage*: T1 hyperintense

Note: Unstable plaques with fibrous cap and outer wall (due to vasa vasorum) can enhance on postcontrast images.

High-risk features:
- *Intraplaque hemorrhage*: Intraplaque hemorrhage (IPH) is associated with symptoms and is a predictor of ischemic stroke.[10,11] IPH by VWI in carotid plaques appears as T1 hyperintensity within the plaque on precontrast T1 WI.
- *Can degree of enhancement predict if a plaque is likely to be the culprit?* In VWI, the atherosclerotic plaque has characteristic features of eccentric wall thickening and enhancement in most cases. Additional T2-weighted imaging T2 hyperintensity in the low-intensity lumen represents the fibrous capsule of the lipid core of the plaque (high levels of cholesterol and cholesterol esters but not triglycerides) and plays an important role in differentiating pathology. When the fibrous capsule breaks, the plaque contents are exposed and demonstrate heterogenous signal intensity on the T2 WI sequence.

The degree of enhancement can be graded on a scale of 0–2 compared to the enhancement of the pituitary stalk. Grade 0 or no enhancement means that the plaque is unlikely to be the cause of stroke, whereas grade 2 enhancement indicates that the plaque is likely to be the cause.

> **Pearl**
> Intracranial atherosclerotic disease (ICAD) plaque enhancement persists for up to 4–8 weeks.

NONATHEROSCLEROTIC DISEASES

Central Nervous System Vasculitis

Central nervous system (CNS) vasculitis[12-15] is usually diagnosed by conventional angiography with nonspecific findings including lumen abnormalities and stenosis.

Pathology

All three layers of the wall are involved namely intima, media, and adventitia. There

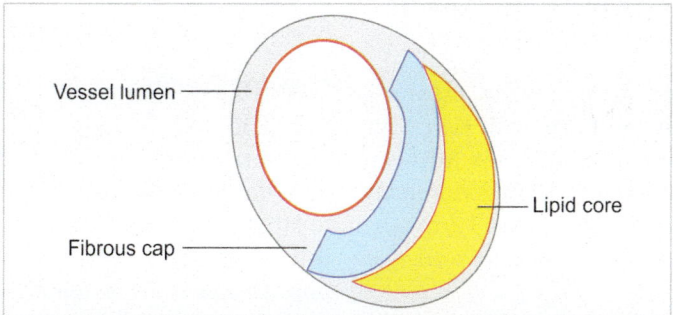

FIG. 4: Diagrammatic representation of the plaque content.

is narrowing of the lumen, while the diameter of the artery remains relatively unchanged. There is increased endothelial permeability and leakage of contrast agent from the lumen into the arterial wall, probably related to the vasa vasorum. The enhancement extends beyond the outer membrane into the periadventitial tissue and persists for a longer time whereas in atherosclerosis the wall enhancement diminishes after 4 weeks.

Imaging Findings

On VW MRI, CNS vasculitis appears as diffuse concentric wall thickening and enhancement in most patients or eccentric thickening and enhancement in a minority of patients. The enhancement pattern in CNS vasculitis usually persists for a long time, with a median duration of 7 months or more.[16]

Clinical Relevance

The MR VWI can potentially be used with high accuracy to diagnose biopsy intracranial inflammatory vessels, predict disease activity, treat and assess therapeutic response. In certain cases, VW MRI serves as a useful tool to differentiate vasculitis from other vessel wall pathologies.

> **Key pearls**
> - Concentric and grade 2 enhancement
> - Enhancement persists for long >7 months.
> - Enhancement does not correlate with disease activity.
> - Enhancement extends beyond the outer membrane into the periadventitial tissue.

In a case of arteriopathy strongly suspected due to vasculitis with non concentric enhancement on MRI, VW MRI can demonstrate juxtaluminal T2 hyperintensity suggesting ICAD. Juxtaluminal T2 hyperintensity suggests fibrous cap and the etiology is ICAD.

Reversible Cerebral Vasoconstriction Syndrome

Reversible cerebral vasoconstriction syndrome (RCVS) diagnostic criteria[17] include:
- Documented multifocal segmental cerebral artery vasospasm on angiography, MRA, or CTA
- Severe acute headache, with or without additional neurologic signs or symptoms
- Vascular reversible angiographic abnormalities within 12 weeks of onset or on postmortem examination to rule out inflammation, intracranial atherosclerosis, or aneurysmal subarachnoid hemorrhage

Reversible cerebral vasoconstriction syndrome has overlapping clinical and imaging features with CNS vasculitis.[15] Differential diagnosis between RCVS and CNS vasculitis is important because of differences in clinical course and treatment; RCVS is treated with follow-up or possibly calcium channel blockers, whereas CNS vasculitis is treated with steroids and Immunosuppression. Recent studies have shown that features of vessel wall in RCVS are different from those in CNS vasculitis, wherein RCVS usually shows concentric wall thickening with very little or mild enhancement, with complete disappearance of wall thickening in recurrent HR-VWI **(Table 2)**.[16]

Pathology

In RCVS, the media layer of the artery is hypertrophied by approximately 500 times.

Imaging Findings

The HR-VWI reveals multiple areas of concentric thickening of the vessel wall with little or no enhancement, corresponding to areas of lumen narrowing. Both wall thickening and lumen narrowing should improve markedly on follow-up imaging.

> **Key pearls (RCVS)**
> - Media is hypertrophied
> - No enhancement

Moyamoya Disease

Moyamoya disease (MMD) is a rare cerebrovascular disease characterized by progressive stenosis of the distal ICA or its proximal main trunk and an abnormal vasculature around the occluded or stenosed artery.[21] The diagnosis of MMD needs to be differentiated from ICAD, and VW-MRI plays an important tool in this regard.

Imaging Findings

In VWI, diffuse concentric signal enhancement represents hyperproliferation of wall components, and diffuse wall thinning represents contraction of the tunica media.[19] Wall enhancement is uncommon, but if present is grade 1.

TABLE 2: Comparison between MR attributes of ICAD, vasculitis, and RCVS.[18-20]

Attribute	ICAD	Vasculitis	RCVS
T2 hyperintensity	Present (80%)	Absent	Absent
T1 wall thickness	Eccentric (90%)	Circumferential (77%)	Circumferential (50%) Absent (30%)
Contrast intensity	Grade 1 (60%) > Grade 2	Grade 2 (60%) > Grade 1	Grade 0 (81%) > Grade 1
Contrast pattern	D>H>F	D	D

Note: Diffuse enhancement (D) was defined as complete enhancement of the lesion, heterogeneous (H) as incomplete lesion enhancement, and focal enhancement (F) was defined as a point or short linear region of lesion enhancement.
(ICAD: intracranial atherosclerotic disease; RCVS: reversible cerebral vasoconstriction syndrome)

Pathology

Intima is hypertrophied, media is thinned outer, thickness remains almost same, negatively remodeled. The pathogenesis of arterial stenosis in atherosclerosis and MMD is fundamentally different. Patients with MMD, regardless of symptoms and stage, have concentric thickening in the distal ICA and MCA with negative remodeling, while patients with ICAD have eccentric thickening and positive remodeling. Wall thickness is slightly increased in MMD but significantly increased in atherosclerosis; T2 signal intensity appears uniform in MMD, whereas patients with ICAD show heterogeneous T2 signal intensity in the vessel wall **(Tables 3 and 4 and Figs. 5 and 6)**.

ANEURYSM

Vessel wall MRI can be used to assess the risk of impending rupture or in case of multiple aneurysms, determining the ruptured aneurysm. CAWE (circumferential aneurysm wall enhancement) includes thin and thick circumferential enhancement and excludes focal eccentric enhancement of the aneurysmal wall.

The score is 0 for no or suspected focal micro enhancement, 1 for focal thick (>1 mm) enhancement, and 2 for thin (maximum thickness ≤ 1 mm) CAWE, or grade 3 for thick (maximum thickness >1 mm) CAWE.[23]

TABLE 3: Comparison between MR attributes of Moyamoya disease and atherosclerosis.[22]

Attribute	Moyamoya	Atherosclerosis
Outer diameter (mm)	2.01	3.31 (↑)
Wall thickness (mm)	0.39	1.64 (↑)
Homogenous signal	83% (↑)	32%

TABLE 4: Comparison between MRI findings various vessel wall pathologies.

	ICAD	Moyamoya	Vasculitis	RCVS
Shape	Eccentric	Concentric	Concentric (sometimes eccentric)	Concentric
Distribution	Any artery	Terminal ICA/ proximal MCA and ACA	Medium to small size vessels	Medium to small size vessels
VW MRI	T2 hyperintense/ heterogenous fibrous cap	–	–	–
Contrast enhancement	Depends on stage (+++ to +)	++/+	Depends on stage (+++ to –)	Depends on stage (+ to –)
Remodeling	Positive/Negative	Negative	–	–
Other features	Intraplaque hemorrhage (T1 hyperintensity)	Basal collaterals	Exclusive diagnosis	Exclusive diagnosis
Follow-up (resolution)	<30%	Progressive	Resolution with medication	Spontaneous reversibility

(ACA: anterior cerebral artery; ICA: internal carotid artery; ICAD: intracranial atherosclerotic disease; MCA: middle cerebral artery; RCVS: reversible cerebral vasoconstriction syndrome)

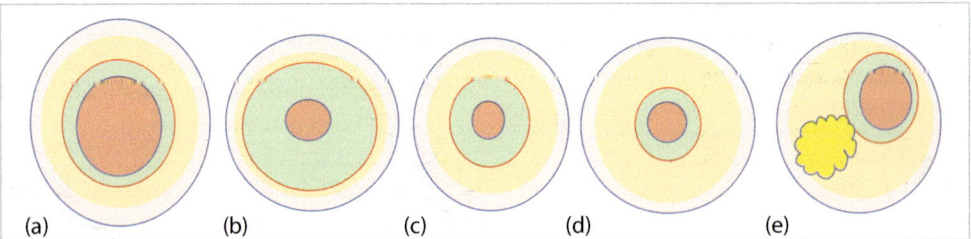

FIG. 5: The histological variation between various steno-occlusive diseases.
(a) Normal intracranial arterial wall consists of intima, internal elastic lamina (green), tunica media (yellow), and adventitia with no or scant vasa vasorum (pink).
(b) Moyamoya disease causes a markedly atrophic tunica media and intimal proliferation resulting in negative remodeling and a narrowed lumen
(c) Vasculitis causes circumferential transmural inflammatory change and areas of wall destruction such as interrupted internal elastic lamina with negative remodeling.
(d) Reversible cerebral vasoconstriction syndrome (RCVS) causes constricted tunica media with narrow lumen and no inflammation.
(e) Atherosclerotic plaque commonly narrows the lumen, but can also eccentrically increase the total diameter of the artery-positive remodeling.

The circumferential pattern of thick (>1 mm) grade 3 wall enhancement shows the highest specificity for unstable aneurysms. Thus, the absence of wall enhancement is a strong predictor of aneurysm stability. This limits the risk of exposing patients with truly stable aneurysms to treatment-related morbidity and mortality.

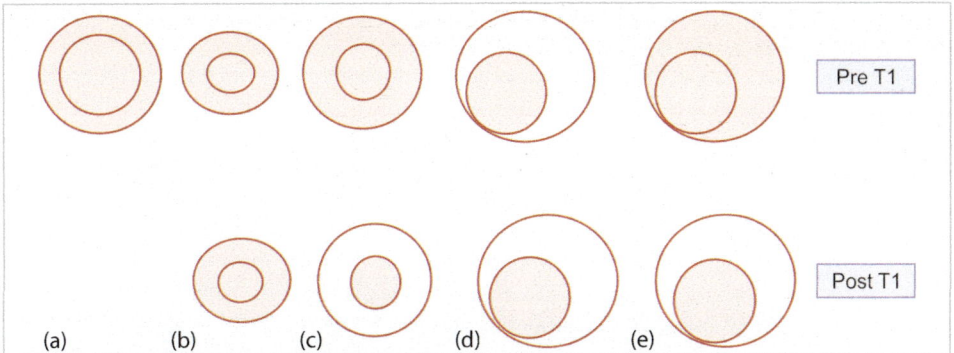

FIG. 6: The MRI VW enhancement pattern of between various steno-occlusive diseases.
(a) Normal intracranial arterial wall
(b) Moyamoya disease negatively remodeled with no or mild enhancement.
(c) Vasculitis causes circumferential enhancement involving all layers.
(d) Intramural dissection shows precontrast T1 hyperintensity suggestive of intramural hematoma.
(e) Atherosclerotic disease showing positive remodeling with eccentric postcontrast T1 enhancement.

■ PITFALLS OF VESSEL WALL MAGNETIC RESONANCE IMAGING

- *Slow flow*: Incomplete signal suppression around the lumen can mimic thickening or enlargement of the vessel wall. Factors predisposing to such artifacts include recurrent or slow flow in aneurysm, slow flow in dilated arteries, and retrograde filling of branching arteries through leptomeningeal collateral vessels during proximal artery occlusion.[24]
- *Vasa vasorum*: In patients with various intracranial artery diseases, vasa vasorum may normally be seen in the proximal intracranial arteries.[1,22]
- Vein-enhancing vein adjacent to an artery may mimic arterial wall enhancement; this can usually be avoided with careful multiplanar examination of VW-MR images and comparison with MR angiography.
- *Effect of thromboembolism and thrombectomy on the arterial wall*: Mechanical thrombectomy can result in concentric wall thickening and enhancement of the intracranial artery wall, mimicking VW-MRI findings in primary arteritis. Similar arterial wall abnormalities are also seen in patients treated with medical therapy alone, but less frequently.

■ CONCLUSION

Addition of vessel wall MRI to routine luminal imaging improved the diagnostic accuracy significantly in patients with focal arteriopathy. It further allows the endovascular interventionists to determine the procedural risk by evaluating remodeling pattern and plaque quadrant. Pearls provided in our chapter will help overcome misinterpretations on vessel wall MRI.

CASES

CASE 1

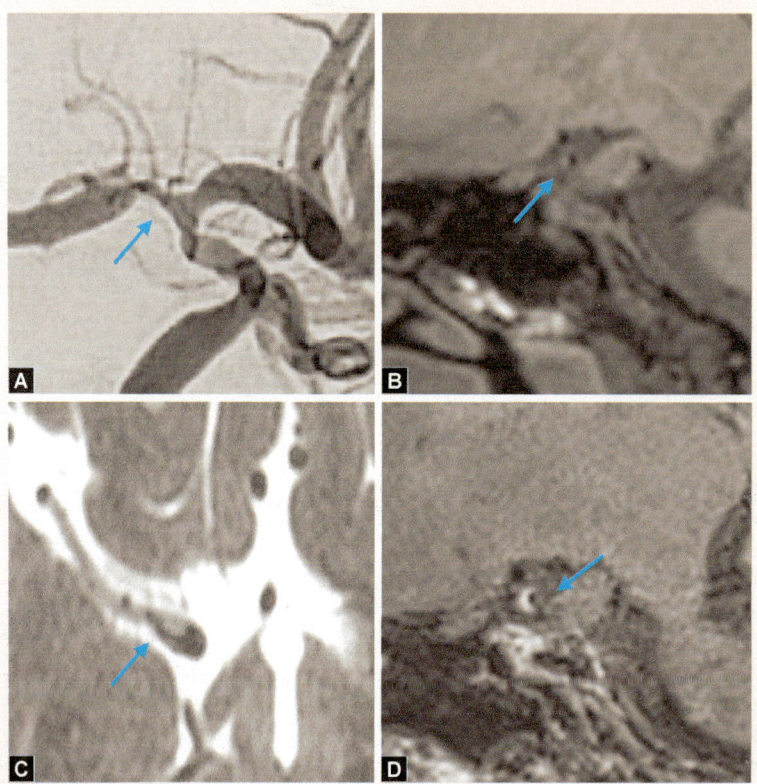

Imaging findings in ICAD:
A. DSA right ICA angiogram shows stenosis at the distal ICA segment and M1 origin (arrowhead).
B. MRI BRAIN sagittal T1WI precontrast shows preserved lumen with small T1 hyperintense foci within the vessel wall suggesting IPH (arrowhead).
C. MRI BRAIN axial T2WI shows T2 hyperintense fibrous cap within the M1 stenotic segment (arrowhead).
D. MRI BRAIN sagittal T1WI postcontrast shows eccentric wall enhancement (arrowhead)

CHAPTER 9: Misinterpretations in Vessel Wall Magnetic Resonance Imaging: Essential Insights   107

CASE 2

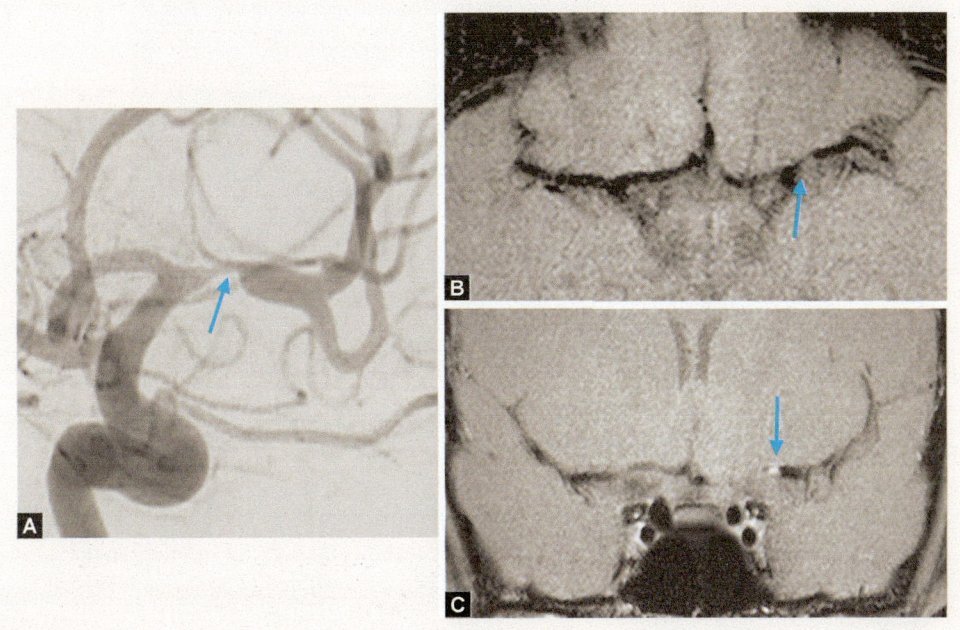

A 37-year-old female with right-sided weakness:
A. DSA- left ICA angiogram AP projection with eccentric stenosis at the left M1 MCA.
B. MRI VW- T1 noncontrast image with left M1 MCA eccentric stenosis.
C. MRI VW- T1 postcontrast coronal image with left M1 MCA plaque enhancement.
Diagnosis-intracranial atheerosclerotic disease (ICAD)

CASE 3

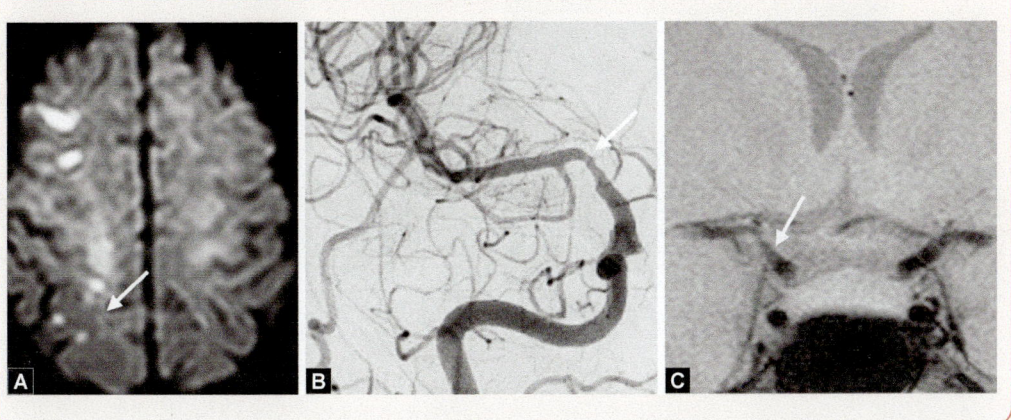

Continued

Continued

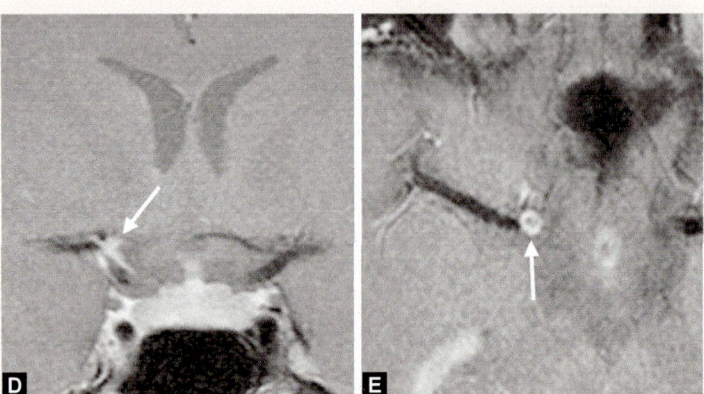

A 22-year-old female with family h/o Fabry's disease, complaints of cataract and skin disease with right hemispheric stroke:

A. MRI: Axial DWI image shows right MCA watershed stroke.
B. DSA: Right CCA angiogram AP view shows stenosis of the right distal ICA and M1 MCA origin.
C. MRI VW: Precontrast T1 coronal image shows stenosis of the distal ICA with wall thickening.
D. MRI VW: Postcontrast T1 coronal image shows enhancement of the distal ICA wall thickening with narrowed lumen.
E. MRI VW: Postcontrast T1 axial image shows concentric enhancement of distal ICA with wall thickening and negative remodeling.

Diagnosis-Vasculitis

CASE 4

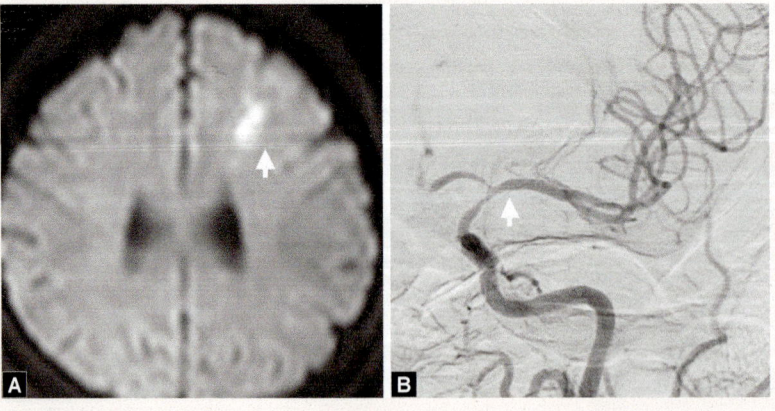

Continued

CHAPTER 9: Misinterpretations in Vessel Wall Magnetic Resonance Imaging: Essential Insights

Continued

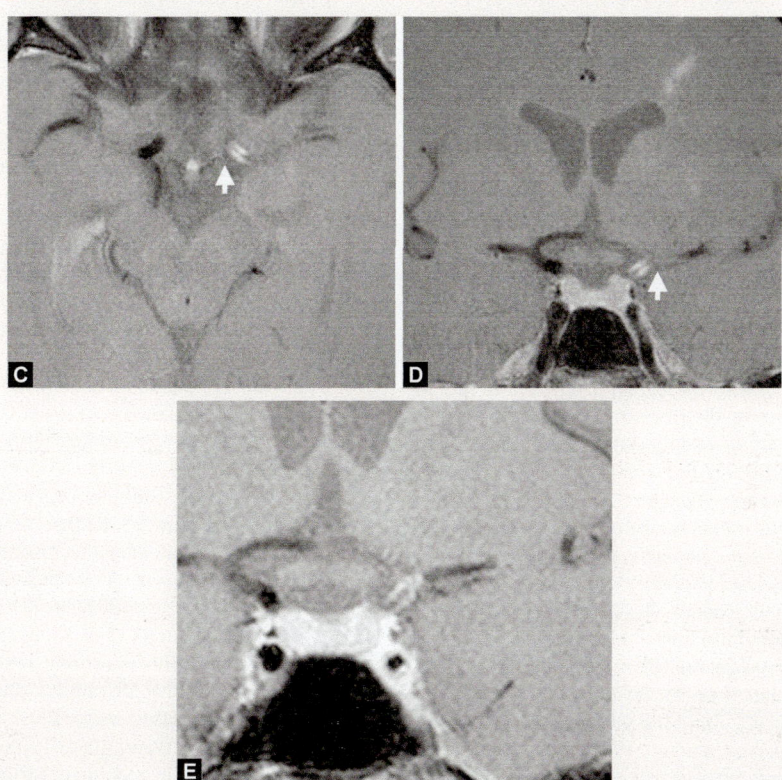

A 35-year-old female with right-sided weakness, no underlying illness:

A. MRI: Axial DWI image shows left ACA infarct.

B. DSA: Left CCA angiogram AP view shows stenosis of the left terminal ICA, M1 MCA origin and A1 ACA origin.

C. MRI VW: Postcontrast T1 axial image shows stenosis of the terminal ICA with wall thickening and concentric enhancement.

D. MRI VW: Postcontrast T1 coronal image shows enhancement of the terminal ICA wall thickening with narrowed lumen and negative remodeling.

E. Vasculitis 9 months follow-up MRI VW: Postcontrast T1 coronal image shows persistent enhancement of the terminal ICA wall thickening with narrowed lumen following diagnosis of vasculitis.

REFERENCES

1. Portanova A, Hakakian N, Mikulis DJ, Virmani R, Abdalla WM, Wasserman BA. Intracranial vasa vasorum: insights and implications for imaging. Radiology. 2013;267(3):667-79.

2. Aydin F. Do human intracranial arteries lack vasa vasorum? A comparative immunohistochemical study of intracranial and systemic arteries. Acta Neuropathol. 1998;96(1):22-8.

3. Connolly Jr ES, Huang J, Goldman JE, Holtzman RN. Immunohistochemical detection of intracranial vasa vasorum: a human autopsy study. Neurosurgery. 1996;38(4):789-93.
4. Takaba M, Endo S, Kurimoto M, Kuwayama N, Nishijima M, Takaku A. Vasa vasorum of the intracranial arteries. Acta Neurochirurgica. 1998;140:411-6.
5. Libby P, Ridker PM, Maseri A. Inflammation and atherosclerosis. Circulation. 2002;105(9):1135-43.
6. Virmani R, Kolodgie FD, Burke AP, Farb A, Schwartz SM. Lessons from sudden coronary death: a comprehensive morphological classification scheme for atherosclerotic lesions. Arterioscler Thromb Vasc Biol. 2000;20(5):1262-75.
7. Xu WH, Li ML, Gao S, Ni J, Zhou LX, Yao M, et al. Plaque distribution of stenotic middle cerebral artery and its clinical relevance. Stroke. 2011;42(10):2957-9.
8. Huang B, Yang WQ, Liu XT, Liu HJ, Li PJ, Lu HK. Basilar artery atherosclerotic plaques distribution in symptomatic patients: a 3.0 T high-resolution MRI study. Eur J Radiol. 2013;82(4):e199-203.
9. Bharadvaj BK, Mabon RF, Giddens DP. Steady flow in a model of the human carotid bifurcation. Part I—flow visualization. J Biomech. 1982;15(5):349-62.
10. Saam T, Hatsukami TS, Takaya N, Chu B, Underhill H, Kerwin WS, et al. The vulnerable, or high-risk, atherosclerotic plaque: noninvasive MR imaging for characterization and assessment. Radiology. 2007;244(1):64-77.
11. Zhao X, Underhill HR, Zhao Q, Cai J, Li F, Oikawa M, et al. Discriminating carotid atherosclerotic lesion severity by luminal stenosis and plaque burden: a comparison utilizing high-resolution magnetic resonance imaging at 3.0 Tesla. Stroke. 2011;42(2):347-53.
12. Aoki S, Hayashi N, Abe O, Shirouzu I, Ishigame K, Okubo T, et al. Radiation-induced arteritis: thickened wall with prominent enhancement on cranial MR images—report of five cases and comparison with 18 cases of moyamoya disease. Radiology. 2002;223(3):683-8.
13. Saam T, Habs M, Pollatos O, Cyran C, Pfefferkorn T, Dichgans M, et al. High-resolution black-blood contrast-enhanced T1 weighted images for the diagnosis and follow-up of intracranial arteritis. Brit J Radiol. 2010;83(993):e182-4.
14. Pfefferkorn T, Linn J, Habs M, Opherk C, Cyran C, Ottomeyer C, et al. Black blood MRI in suspected large artery primary angiitis of the central nervous system. J Neuroimag. 2013;23(3):379-83.
15. Mossa-Basha M, Hwang WD, De Havenon A, Hippe D, Balu N, Becker KJ, et al. Multicontrast high-resolution vessel wall magnetic resonance imaging and its value in differentiating intracranial vasculopathic processes. Stroke. 2015;46(6):1567-73.
16. Obusez EC, Hui F, Hajj-Ali RA, Cerejo R, Calabrese LH, Hammad T, et al. High-resolution MRI vessel wall imaging: spatial and temporal patterns of reversible cerebral vasoconstriction syndrome and central nervous system vasculitis. Am J Neuroradiol. 2014;35(8):1527-32.
17. Calabrese LH, Dodick DW, Schwedt TJ, Singhal AB. Narrative review: reversible cerebral vasoconstriction syndromes. Ann Intern Med. 2007;146(1):34-44.
18. Mossa-Basha M, Shibata DK, Hallam DK, De Havenon A, Hippe DS, Becker KJ, et al. Added value of vessel wall magnetic resonance imaging for differentiation of nonocclusive intracranial vasculopathies. Stroke. 2017;48(11):3026-33.
19. Ryoo S, Cha J, Kim SJ, Choi JW, Ki CS, Kim KH, et al. High-resolution magnetic resonance wall imaging findings of Moyamoya disease. Stroke. 2014;45(8):2457-60.
20. Yuan M, Liu ZQ, Wang ZQ, Li B, Xu I I, Xiao XL. High-resolution MR imaging of the arterial wall in moyamoya disease. Neurosci Lett. 2015;584:77-82.
21. Scott RM, Smith ER. Moyamoya disease and moyamoya syndrome. N Engl J Med. 2009;360(12):1226-37.
22. Aoki S, Shirouzu I, Sasaki Y, Okubo T, Hayashi N, Machida T, et al. Enhancement of the intracranial arterial wall at MR imaging: relationship to cerebral atherosclerosis. Radiology. 1995;194(2):477-81.
23. Edjlali M, Guédon A, Ben Hassen W, Boulouis G, Benzakoun J, Rodriguez-Régent C, et al. Circumferential thick enhancement at vessel wall MRI has high specificity for intracranial aneurysm instability. Radiology. 2018;289(1):181-7.
24. Hui FK, Zhu X, Jones SE, Uchino K, Bullen JA, Hussain MS, et al. Early experience in high-resolution MRI for large vessel occlusions. J Neurointerv Surg. 2015;7(7):509-16.

CHAPTER 10

Beyond Antithrombotic in Secondary Prevention of Stroke

Debsiash Hota, Biplab Das, Somalin Satapathy

ABSTRACT

The purpose of this chapter emphasis on review of holistic approach of stroke prevention with respect to latest guidelines. Antithrombotics are very essential in preventing stroke recurrence but various other factors have also significant impact on management of stroke prevention.

Stroke is considered as third leading cause of mortality worldwide. Over the last decade, there is significant rise in number of stroke attributed to various factors including COVID, pollution, sedentary lifestyle, and unhealthy diet habits. Prevention of stroke is very vital and it has a significant effect on health and welfare of population even if very effective acute treatment available.

Hyperacute management stroke is changing its landscape in long-term prognosis. In the other hand, stroke is largely preventable. The mainstays focus on medical management including antihypertensive, proper glycemic control, lipid-lowering agent, and antithrombotic but in current era of evidence-based medicine, there is larger scope of intravascular intervention for long-term stroke prevention. Identification of exact etiology plays an vital role for tailored individualized treatment. Largely, community participation with stroke awareness and behavioral intervention are gaining upper hand on stroke prevention.

Keywords: ICAD, ECAD, CAS, CEA, OSA, PFO, TCD, TEE.

■ INTRODUCTION[1]

Stroke is defined as a sudden onset focal neurological deficit that is attributable to a vascular cause. Stroke is a clinical event and brain imaging is used to confirm the diagnosis. The clinical presentation of cerebrovascular event is highly variable due to complex anatomy of brain and its vascular supply. Stroke is broadly classified into ischemic and hemorrhagic stroke. Ischemic stroke usually manifests as group of clinical features ascribable to certain areas of brain supplied by a single vascular region. Intracranial hemorrhage produces signs and symptoms due to mass effect or intracranial pressure which may not be confined to a vascular territory.

■ EPIDEMIOLOGY[2-5]

Stroke is one of the leading causes of morbidity and mortality in India. The estimated incidence is 105–152 per lakh population and prevalence ranged from 45 to 559 per lakh.

In the last decade, there has been an increase in the incidence of stroke in younger population and even more in post-COVID era attributed to prothrombotic state after COVID infection and vaccination. Out of all strokes, 85% are ischemic, 13% are hemorrhagic, and 2% are subarachnoid hemorrhage. Approximately one-third of patients experience warning transient ischemic attack (TIA) before stroke. Annual stroke recurrence was almost 8.7% five decades back; now it has come down to below 5% with significant effort of secondary prevention. Approximately 90.5% of the global stroke burdens are due to modifiable risk factors. The majority of risk factors are blood pressure, diet, physical inactivity, smoking, and abdominal obesity. Out of all ischemic strokes, 17% are attributed to atrial fibrillation (AF), 4% due to carotid disease, rest 64% are due to other specific causes. In case of hemorrhagic stroke, 7% are hypertensive bleeds, 4% are aneurysmal subarachnoid bleeds, and rest are due to unknown causes.

■ STROKE CLASSIFICATION[6-9]

Clinicoradilogical stroke classification is given in **Table 1**.

■ PATHOPHYSIOLOGY OF STROKE[10,11]

Mechanism of stroke whether atherothrombosis or embolization from proximal artery or heart is very vital for management and prevention of stroke **(Fig. 1)**.

■ STROKE TERMINOLOGY

Type of cerebral circulation failure are given in **Table 2**.

■ GUIDELINE FOR SECONDARY STROKE PREVENTION[12]

For strategical approach, it should be divided into broadly four categories:
1. Diagnostic evaluation for secondary stroke prevention
2. Addressing vascular risk factors
3. Etiological management
4. System of care for secondary prevention

■ DIAGNOSTIC EVALUATION OF STROKE[13,14]

Patient presented with sign and symptoms of acute stroke should undergo urgent

TABLE 1: Classification of stroke.

Stroke type	Description
Lacunar	CT/MR showing cortical or subcortical infract measuring <1.5 cm
Small vessel disease	CT/MR showing mostly subcortical lesion of size <1.5 cm without concomitant cortical infract
Cardioembolic	Infract attributed to occlusion of arterial territories with embolus sourced from heart. There is always involvement of more than one vascular territory
Cryptogenic	Imaging and clinical confirmation of stroke without a confirmed source on extended routine evaluation protocol. Can be lacunar or larger in size and nonembolic in nature
ESUS	Imaging and clinical confirmation of stroke which are nonlacunar and embolic pattern without source being identified
Large artery atherosclerosis	Ischemic stroke in vascular territory with major intra- or extracranial stenosis on imaging. Size of lesion >1.5 cm with either cortical or subcortical or brainstem or cerebellar involvement

(ESUS: embolic stroke of undetermined source)

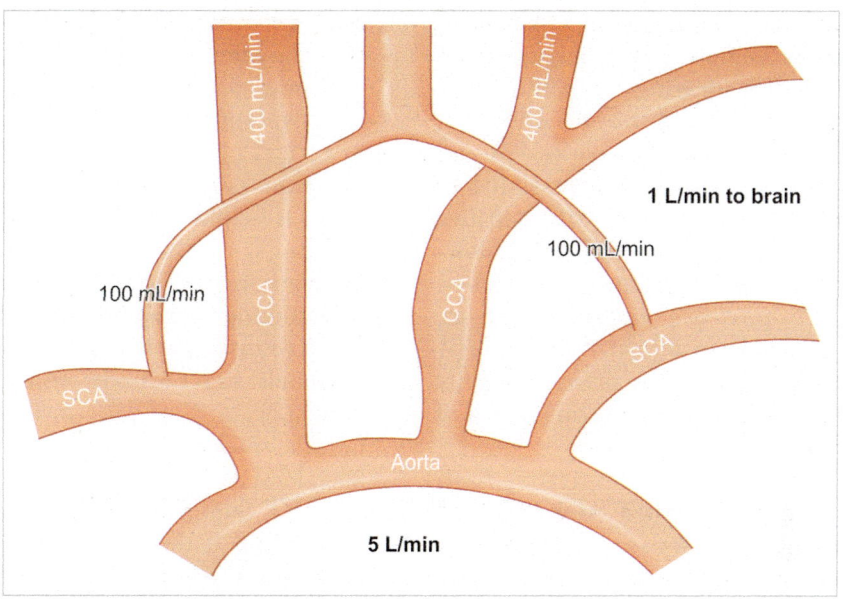

FIG. 1: Stroke pathophysiology.

TABLE 2: Terminologies.

Terminology	Description
Cerebral ischemia	Due to reduction in blood flow that sustains longer than few seconds
Transient ischemic attack (TIA)	A condition wherein all neurological signs and symptoms resolve within 24 hours without evidence of brain infarction on imaging
Syncope	It is generalized reduction in cerebral blood flow due to systemic hypotension of any cause. If low cerebral blood persists longer
Hypoperfusion infract	Low blood flow to brain due to circulatory failure caused by the failing of the heart's pumping action (heart attack) or severe stenosis in artery that leads to border zone infraction

imaging to identify type of stroke and expedite reperfusion therapy based on standard protocol. Simultaneously patient should be evaluated in detailed to recognize to possible etiology of stroke and prioritize treatment for secondary prevention. Sometimes confirmation of stroke might require follow-up imaging as noncontrast CT has poor sensitivity for hyperacute and small infract. The risk of recurrent stroke in short term and long term depends upon stroke mechanism. The risk of stroke within first 3 month is about 5% but can vary as per stroke pathophysiology. We have listed below some basic and advanced diagnostic test tailored as per patient clinical status and imaging. Patient with stroke should undergo required diagnostic test for deciding optimal strategies within 48 hours of stroke symptoms.

- *Electrocardiogram (ECG)*: It is a basic and noninvasive test to identify AF as risk factor for stroke. It is also helpful to diagnose acute myocardial infarction which can occur simultaneously in about 3% of patients.
- *Brain imaging*: This is the first imaging to be performed to exclude hemorrhage. About 15–25% patient with clinical symptom of stroke will have alternate diagnosis with the help of imaging. On

contrary, 13% of patients with symptoms thought to be nonstroke will have stroke diagnosis on imaging. In multicentric study, focal nonmotor and nonspeech neurological deficit with positive diffusion restriction has six times increase risk of recurrent stroke at 1 year. MRI negative stroke has prevalence of 2% but follow-up MRI can pick up diffusion restriction mostly in posterior circulation stroke. It is advisable to repeat CT scan after 24–72 hours after stroke onset to identify any hemorrhagic transformation and midline shift.

- *Vascular imaging*: Patients with symptomatic carotid stenosis are candidates for revascularization, it is essential to screen for any stenosis in anterior or posterior circulation. Noninvasive batteries of test available are carotid Doppler, MR angiography, and CT angiography in increasing order of sensitivity, the gold standard test being digital subtraction angiography. Some centers are also doing vessel wall imaging for identifying character of unstable plaque like intraplaque hemorrhage.
- *Routine blood parameter*: Recommended batteries of test include FBS, HbA1c, renal function test, liver function test, PT-INR, aPTT, and lipid profile.
- *Special blood tests*: This type of test needs to be performed if there is clinical suspicion with younger age population. Test includes APLA panel, vasculitis profile, thrombophilia profile, and homocysteine level. Yield of hypercoagulable state is low for patient of >50 years. In special cases, toxicology screening should be done at presentation as cocaine used within 24 hours increases stroke by six times. In recent studies, monogenic causes of stroke were 7%.
- *Basic cardiological test*: Echocardiography is very essential to confirming the stroke etiology. It can identify cardiomegaly, LA enlargement, ejection fraction, atrial myxoma, patent foramen ovale, and infective endocarditis. Transthoracic is better for LV thrombus and routine studies but transesophageal echocardiogram (TEE) is helpful for LA thrombus, aortic atheroma, cardiac tumors, and patent foramen ovale (PFO). TEE will be helpful in changing management of stroke in about 15% patients with prior categorized as embolic stroke of undetermined source (ESUS).
- *Cardiac rhythm monitoring*: Holter study for at least 24 hours is essential to identify silent AF. Sometimes longer monitoring is required if there is strong imaging indication and rest evaluation is negative. Repeated Holter in patient with age >60 years with recent stroke increases chance of AF detection in about 14%.
- *Transcranial Doppler (TCD)*: It is one of the very informative and noninvasive tests to detect right to left shunt which is due to PFO. Bubble study for PFO has sensitivity of 96.1%. TCD is also useful in identifying micro emboli.

VASCULAR RISK FACTOR MANAGEMENT[15-18]

Majority of risk factors of stroke are modifiable:
- *Diet and nutrition*:[19] Food is one of essential components of stroke prevention strategy. Patient with stroke should be advised for proper healthy diet. There are two categories of diet for risk management, one being Mediterranean diet which relies on monosaturated fat, plant-based foods, and fish consumption with extra virgin oil or nut supplementation and the being low sodium consumption at least reduced by 1 g/d up to 2.5 g/d, which is very effective for cardiovascular disease. Many studies

support protective effects of regular fish intake, high fruit, and vegetable consumption along high-fiber diet. There are major long-term hazardous effects of fried food, added fats, processed meats, and sugar-sweetened beverages which can be associated with 40% increased risk of stroke. Overall, high K^+ and low Na^+ are associated with lower stroke rates. Low salt diet is associated with greater reduction of systolic blood pressure (SBP) **(Table 3)**.

- *Physical activity*:[20] Regular physical activity positively affects stroke risk factors. It has a very vital role in onset stroke severity, enhanced endothelial function, and reduced platelet aggregation and fibrinogen levels. Sitting >4 h/day is a risk factor for cardiovascular disease. Increase in moderate to vigorous intensity exercise has positive impact in vascular risk factors. The recommended physical activity is about 40 minutes session in each day for at least 3–4 days per week of moderate to vigorous activity but practically it is not possible for all stroke survivor. So, it should be customized as per tolerance, stage of recovery, specific impairments, and available social support. Studies advised for minimum 10 minutes aerobic activity 4 times a week or vigorous intensity aerobic exercise for 20 minutes twice a week. Physical activity also has favorable impact on aerobic fitness, mobility, functional balance, and most importantly on behavioral change. Some of patients with stroke may have substantial weakness, impaired cognition, and altered perception which can be barrier for active participation. This type of patient should undergo robotic-assisted physical activity and use of adaptive equipment along skill personnel can help to prevail over barrier to participation. For nonambulatory patients, exercise program is safe and feasible. Another study showed sitting with 3 minutes bout of light exercise or standing every 30 minutes decreased SBP by 3.5–5 mm Hg.

- *Smoking cessation*:[21] Active smoking is a potent, independent, and dose-dependent risk factor for ischemic stroke and silent brain infarction. Tobacco is an additive behavior and cessation is difficult. Long-term mortality is associated with persistent smoking and same enhances recurrent stroke by two times. As per expert opinion, there is trend of increased smoking cessation in stroke survivors. Passive smoking also carries substantial risk of recurrent stroke.

- *Substance abuse*:[22] Alcohol consumption of >30 drinks/month or binge drink of >5/day at least once per month is associated with high risk of recurrent stroke. Alcohol use causes chronic relapsing brain disease with compulsive drinking and negative emotional state. There is

TABLE 3: Diet categories for risk management.

Mediterranean diet	DASH diet
High monosaturated/saturated fat ratio	Limited saturated fat and cholesterol
High intake of plant-based foods (fruit, vegetables, and legumes)	More fruit, vegetables, and legumes
High intake of whole grains, cereals	High whole grains
Increased intake of fish	
Low consumption of meat and no processed meat	Limited meats
Low-to-moderate red wine	
Moderate consumption of milk and dairy products	Fat free/low fat dairy
No soda drinks, pastries, sweets, bakery products, and spread fats	Limited sweets/sweetened beverages, salts

certain gender inequality of stroke risk with respect to ethanol consumption as evident by consuming more than two drinks a day for male carries equal risk of one drink in female. Other substances like amphetamines, cocaine, or intravenous drugs also carry very high risk of recurrent stroke which can be addressed by behavioral intervention on repeated basis.

- *Hypertension*:[23] It is one of the very potential yet neglected risk factors for all cardiovascular event. On an average, one-third populations are hypertensive, of which half of them are not taking it seriously and rest half mismanaged. Ideal target for blood pressure remains SBP 120–130 mm Hg/diastolic blood pressure (DBP) 80–90 mm Hg. Choices of antihypertensives as first line are diuretics, angiotensin-converting enzyme (ACE) inhibitors, and angiotensin receptor blocker (ARB) as they have other long-term positive impact on heart and kidney. Second-line drug includes calcium channel blocker and beta-blockers. Major hurdles remain on optimal dosing and monitoring of BP on daily basis to avoid any large variability. Sudden uprise can lead to recurrent hemorrhagic stroke or sudden downfall can lead to hypoperfusion infarct. Overall, the magnitude of BP reduction is essential that type of drug used. Sometimes, it is advisable to keep BP on higher level to optimize functioning of collaterals or cross flow in case of near total occlusion of one of the major artery.
- *Hyperlipidemia*:[24] It is one of the most important cause of vascular disease due to its long-term effect on vessel wall. Sedentary lifestyles with high saturated fat and excessive carbohydrates intake will eventually lead to plaque formation in vessel walls which can be flow limiting subsequently. Major studies conducted earlier concluded that ideal goal should be low-density lipoprotein (LDL) < 70 mg/dL to optimal benefit. Patients with stroke having LDL >100 mg/dL should receive at least 80 mg of statin to achieve the target. Compliance to LDL-lowering diet can also reduce level by 10–15%, but moderate-intensity statin and high-intensity statin can effectively reduce level by 30–40% and >50% respectively. Sometimes ezetimibe can be added as first line who not optimally responding to statin only. Ezetimibe use before PCSK9 inhibitor has advantage of safety profile, available in generic form and good synergistic action with statins. Special emphasis should be given to those with intra- or extracranial atherosclerosis on imaging. Patient with high cardiovascular risk taking maximally tolerated dose of both statin and ezetimibe ideally should receive PCSK9 inhibitor like alirocumab and evolocumab. Effectivity of lipid-lowering agents should be assessed at 12-week interval.
- *Hypertriglyceridemia*:[25] One of the independent risk factors associated with recurrent stroke is triglyceride level even if cholesterol level is normal. Patients with stroke or TIA having triglyceride >135 mg/dL should receive extended release niacin and fibrates as initial treatment. High triglyceride level without AF or heart failure should receive icosapent ethyl (IPE) 2 g twice daily to reduce recurrent stroke. With very high TG level (>500 mg/dL), it is better to identify genetic risk along with initiation of very low-fat diet, avoidance of refined carbs and alcohol and intake of omega fatty acid should be followed.
- *Diabetes*:[26] India being diabetic capital should be managed very efficiently to reduce any cardiovascular event. The goal of diabetes control should be individualized based on adverse effect profile, patient preferences to achieve HbA1c of <7 which will beneficial for

preventing micro- and macrovascular complications. Multidimensional care is cornerstone for diabetes control with emphasis not only on medication but also on diet and exercise. Patient with prediabetes/impaired glucose tolerance should be advised for lifestyle modification including weight reduction. Metformin and sulfonylurea are first-line agents along with pioglitazone. About 20% of patients with stroke found to have undiagnosed diabetes but on contrary 30% have prediabetes, and 50% have insulin resistance. In other sense, one out of two with stroke has insulin resistance. Uncontrolled DM on long-term is associated with CNS small vessel disease (SVD) and vascular dementia. It is pivotal to treat hyperglycemia to reduce recurrent stroke and subclinical ischemic changes.

- *Obesity*:[27] In current era, there is increasing burden of obesity which leads to various complication on long run including vascular events. Obesity increases risk of stroke by >50% and is closely linked with dyslipidemia, AF, and elevated BP. The best way to intervene obesity is intense behavioral counseling along with medication and metabolic surgery. Modest loss of weight by 5–10% will have positive impact on further cardiovascular events and glycemic control.
- *Obstructive sleep apnea (OSA)*:[28] OSA is one of the silent risk factors of stroke. There is 10% prevalence of sleep apnea among general population. Sleep apnea is diagnosed by polysomnography which is based on AHI (apnea–hypopnea index). There is increased risk of stroke mortality, hypertension, and AF linked with sleep apnea. Continuous positive airway pressure (CPAP) used as first-line management for OSA along with weight reduction is helpful in sleep-related quality of life and physical functioning.

ETIOLOGICAL APPROACH FOR SECONDARY PREVENTION

Large Artery Atherosclerosis

There are two modalities of treatment from an anatomical point of view.

Intracranial Atherosclerosis[29]

There is increasing evidence of major intracranial atherosclerosis contributing to recurrent stroke. Major studies showed that degree of stenosis is an important predictor of stroke recurrence with a tune of almost 18% chance of recurrence if >70% stenosis noted. However, subset patients with low flow or poor collaterals have even high risk of recurrence. Trials like CHANCE and CLAIR showed evidence of dual antiplatelet to be used for ICAD. Consensus regarding duration of DAPT (aspirin + clopidogrel) varies from studies to studies. The standard recommendation is of at least 90 days. Some studies also advised for use ticagrelor 90 mg twice or cilostazol 200 mg with aspirin. Apart from antiplatelets, there is significant role of antihypertensive to achieve target SBP of <140 mm Hg, high-intensity statins, and physical activity. In case of severe stenosis of >70% with progressing symptoms or recurrent TIA even after DAPT/medical failure, there is certain scope of angioplasty alone or stent deployment but such strategies are under robust trial as there is no beneficial role of primary angioplasty established yet. There is also no recommendation of extra intracranial bypass. SAMMPRIS trial and VISSIT trial for anterior circulation and VAST and VIST trial for posterior circulation support best medical management over percutaneous transluminal angioplasty and stenting (PTAS).

Extracranial Atherosclerosis[30]

Atherosclerosis of carotid bulb or ostium of vertebral artery is common among the stroke survivor. In case of recurrent TIA/nondisabling stroke with ipsilateral stenosis of >70%, it is recommended to do carotid revascularization procedure within 2 weeks of acute stroke which can be beneficial for recurrent stroke prevention. Severe stenosis of >70% in asymptomatic side also found to be beneficial from carotid revascularization. CEA (carotid endarterectomy) is preferred over CAS (carotid artery stenting) in majority of study with periprocedural risk of <6%. In situation of ipsilateral symptomatic moderate stenosis of 50–69%, carotid revascularization should be done with CEA. In case of nonsymptomatic moderate stenosis, it is advisable to follow strict medical management composing of antiplatelets, antihypertensives, and lipid-lowering agents. In NASCET and CREST trial, CEA can be performed in >70 years age or within 1 week of index stroke if periprocedural risk is <6%. CAS is indicated with >70% stenosis if there is multiple comorbidities, radiation-induced stenosis, or restenosis after CEA. In case of stenosis <50%, carotid revascularization is not recommended in first instance. In case of posterior circulation, stroke prevalence of extracranial vertebral stenosis is about 10% but recent guidelines do not recommend any angioplasty or stenting rather advisable to follow best medical management.

Aortic arch atherosclerosis: Stroke evaluation is not complete until there is proper evaluation of aortic arch. Aortic arch atheroma is also silent cause of recurrent noncardioembolic stroke which need detailed study either by transesophageal ECHO (TEE) or by MRI TOF angiography. The recommended guidelines are best medical therapy consisting of high-intensity statins with single antiplatelet therapy (SAPT).

Moyamoya Disease[31]

It is an idiopathic steno-occlusive disease of arteries of circle of Willis with abnormal collaterals development in lenticulostriate arteries giving rise to puff of smoke appearance. It has a bimodal distribution with peak in childhood (ischemic) and adulthood (hemorrhagic). The recommendation for recurrent stroke prevention in Moyamoya is surgical revascularization with direct or indirect bypass involving superficial temporal artery with middle cerebral artery and aspirin monotherapy.

Small Vessel Disease[32]

Small vessel disease constitutes 20–30% of all strokes. Hypertensive and diabetes are being notable cause of SVD. Recurrence of SVD varies from 4 to 11% per year. SVD is one of the major contributors of vascular dementia and vascular cognitive impairment. Best medical management is cornerstone for SVD recurrence with monotherapy with aspirin or cilostazol.

Cardioembolism[33]

Atrial Fibrillation

It is one of the major contributors of recurrent stroke. Left atrial appendage is main source of cardioembolism with >90% site of thrombus is found here. Non-vitamin K oral anticoagulants (NOACs) are cornerstone for secondary prevention of stroke but patient will have high risk of bleed or with contraindication for lifelong anticoagulation; it is advisable to consider for percutaneous closure of left atrial appendage with watchman device.

Valvular Heart Disease

Rheumatic heart disease is very prevalent in developing countries. With moderate-to-severe MS, vitamin K antagonist is first-line treatment for stroke prevention with target INR of 2–3. Apart from medication, there is also recommendation for early valve surgery along with optimal medication. One of the less known causes of stroke is infective endocarditis which required full therapeutic course of antibiotics before proceeding for surgery. IE has independent risk of hemorrhagic conversion, mycotic aneurysm, or septic necrotic arteritis.

Left Ventricular Thrombus

Abnormal contractility of left ventricular (LV) apex will eventually lead to blood pooling and subsequent thrombus formation. Patients with recent anterior wall MI are at high risk for LV thrombus formation. The recommendation is of at least 3 month of anticoagulation to reduce stroke recurrence.

Cardiomyopathy

Cardiomyopathy with reduced ejection fraction (EF) has higher incidence of thromboembolism. There is definite role of anticoagulation with warfarin for at least more than 3 month, but in case of LV-assisted device, warfarin should be combined with aspirin.

Patent Foramen Ovale

It is one of the greatest masquerade of recurrent stroke. Diagnosis test is based on clinical suspicion without any known risk factors. Ideal tests that need to be done include TEE and TCD. For large PFO with atrial septal aneurysm it is recommended to undergo transcatheter PFO closure along with long term antiplatelets. Risk of procedural complication showed 4.9% in <60 years versus 10.9% in >60 years.

Congenital Heart Disease and Cardiac Tumors

Rarely, congenital heart disease associated with stroke in young population for which anticoagulation with warfarin is recommended. Primary cardiac tumors are atrial myxoma and fibroelastoma which have 25% chance of embolism.

Dissection[34,35]

Dissection in extracranial vertebral and carotid artery is mostly either traumatic or spontaneous. Artery to artery embolization from intraluminal thrombus is most common mechanism of recurrent stroke. Guideline supports use of either antiplatelet or anticoagulant for 3-month duration. Cases of recurrent stroke and pseudoaneurysm formation who are not responding to optimal medical management should be advised for endovascular stenting.

Hypercoagulable State[36]

Guidelines for management of hypercoagulable state is given in **Table 4**.

Special Conditions Leading to Recurrent Stroke[37]

Guidelines for management of stroke in special situations given in **Table 5**.

TABLE 4: Recommendation for management of hypercoagulable state.

List of parameters	Recommendation
Protein C and S deficiency	Antiplatelet to be considered
Antithrombin III deficiency	
Factor V Leiden mutation	
Antiphospholipid syndrome	• If single antibody positive—consider antiplatelet • If triple antibody positive—consider anticoagulant (warfarin)
Hyperhomocysteinemia	Supplement with B6, B12, and folate

TABLE 5: Recommendation for special conditions.

List of disease	Recommendation
Malignancy	Anticoagulant to be considered with primary treatment of malignancy
Sickle cell disease	Recurrent blood transfusion and hydroxyurea
Vasculitis	High-dose glucocorticoids with steroid sparing agents as immunosuppressants like methotrexate or tocilizumab
Primary CNS angiitis	High-dose steroids + steroid-sparing agent (MMF/rituximab/azathioprine/cyclophosphamide)
MELAS (mitochondrial myopathy, encephalopathy, lactic acidosis, stroke-like episodes)	Oral L-arginine + intravenous L-arginine
Carotid web (thin circumferential shelf like filling defect on carotid bulb)	Antiplatelets + carotid stenting if delayed stasis noted in angiogram
Fibromuscular dysplasia (nonatherosclerotic segmental disease of small and medium size arteries)	Antiplatelets + BP control + lifestyle modification As first line, if not responding, carotid angioplasty with stenting can be considered
Dolichoectasia (fusiform dilatation and tortuosity of vertebrobasilar segment)	Either antiplatelet or anticoagulant is reasonable
ESUS (nonlacunar cryptogenic embolic pattern of stroke)	Anticoagulant like DOAC or ticagrelor may be considered if extensive work-up negative and high recurrence rate

(DOAC: direct oral anticoagulant; ESUS: embolic stroke of undetermined source)

■ SYSTEM OF CARE FOR SECONDARY PREVENTION

For point of discussion and effective intervention, it is subcategorized into three segments.

Health System-based Intervention[38]

In a patient with stroke, outpatient-focused or voluntary hospital-based quality monitoring and improvement program are advised for better compliance to evidence based guidelines. Multidisciplinary team strategy including caregiver, nurses, pharmacists, and physiotherapist should be developed for effective control of modifiable risk factors. Sometimes appropriate triage or customized plan should be initiated for lifestyle modification.

Behavioral Modification[39]

For holistic approach regarding stroke prevention, it is ideal to educate properly in term of stroke literacy, medication compliance, and lifestyle factors. Training regarding self-management tool and motivational interview can be effective for medication adherence. There should be a combined approach for physical activity with behavioral intervention. For disabling stroke after discharge from facility, patient should be advised for adapted cardiac rehabilitation, aerobic activity, and lifestyle modification.

Health Equity[40]

Socioeconomic status has a major impact on stroke recurrence. Addressing social determinants like medication affordability, food insecurity, housing, transportation barrier, manpower barrier, language proficiency, and literacy level is very vital for long-term recovery and stroke prevention. There should be hospital protocol-based screening tool to address major five domains such as nutrition, transportation, utility assistance, interpersonal safety, and housing instability.

■ CONCLUSION

Diagnostic work-up after stroke is cornerstone for establishing stroke etiology and to target optimal management. Management of vascular risk factors like DM, dyslipidemia, hypertension, and smoking cessation remains cornerstone in secondary prevention of stroke. Healthy diet and physical activity are also pivotal in stroke recurrence. Changing behavior with medication adherence required targeted effort at individual level. Antithrombotics are just not enough for achieving target. Specific source of recurrence like extracranial atherosclerosis should intervene within time limit for maximal result. Intracranial atherosclerosis is one of leading cause of stroke recurrence and should be managed optimally with medication. Last not the least, judicious use of antithrombotic is also essential for best results and minimizing complications. Multidimensional holistic team approach is proving difference in long-term outcome.

REFERENCES

1. Hopkinsmedicine.org. (2022). Types of stroke. [online] Available from https://www.hopkinsmedicine.org/health/conditions-and-diseases/stroke/types-of-stroke. [Last accessed August, 2024]
2. Virani SS, Alonso A, Benjamin EJ, Bittencourt MS, Callaway CW, Carson AP, et al. Heart disease and stroke statistics—2020 update: A report from the American Heart Association. Circulation. 2020;141(9);e139-e596.
3. Kleindorfer D, Panagos P, Pancioli A, Khoury J, Kissela B, Woo D, et al. Incidence and short-term prognosis of Transient ischemic attack in a population-based study. Stroke. 2005;36(4):720-3.
4. Benjamin EJ, Blaha MJ, Chiuve SE, Cushman M, Das SR, Deo R, et al. Heart disease and stroke statistics-2017 update: A report from the American heart association. Circulation. 2017;135(10):e146-603.
5. Pandian JD, Sudhan P. Stroke epidemiology and stroke care services in India. J Stroke. 2013;15(3):128-34.
6. Gore M, Bansal K, Khan Suheb MZ, Lui F, Asuncion RMD. (2024). Lacunar Stroke. [online] Available from https://www.ncbi.nlm.nih.gov/books/NBK563216/. [Last accessed August, 2024]
7. Ntaios G. Embolic stroke of undetermined source. J Am Coll Cardiol. 2020;75(3):333-40.
8. Yetman D. (2023). Cryptogenic stroke: Definition, causes, symptoms, treatment. Healthline. [online] Available from https://www.healthline.com/health/stroke/cryptogenic-stroke. [Last accessed August, 2024]
9. Singh A, Bonnell G, De Prey J, Buchwald N, Eskander K, Kincaid KJ, et al. Small-vessel disease in the brain. Am Heart J Plus. 2023;27(100277):100277.
10. Woodruff TM, Thundyil J, Tang S-C, Sobey CG, Taylor SM, Arumugam TV. Pathophysiology, treatment, and animal and cellular models of human ischemic stroke. Mol Neurodegener. 2011;6(1):11.
11. Kuriakose D, Xiao Z. Pathophysiology and treatment of stroke: Present status and future perspectives. Int J Mol Sci. 2020;21(20):7609.
12. Kleindorfer DO, Towfighi A, Chaturvedi S, Cockroft KM, Gutierrez J, Lombardi-Hill D, et al. 2021 guideline for the prevention of stroke in patients with stroke and transient ischemic attack: A guideline from the American heart association/American stroke association. Stroke. 2021;52(7):e364-e467.
13. NHLBI, NIH. (2023). Diagnosis. [online] Available from https://www.nhlbi.nih.gov/health/stroke/diagnosis. [Last accessed August, 2024]
14. Mayoclinic.org. (2024). Stroke. [online] Available from https://www.mayoclinic.org/diseases-conditions/stroke/diagnosis-treatment/drc-20350119. [Last accessed August, 2024]
15. Prabhakaran S, Chong JY. Risk factor management for stroke prevention. Continuum (Minneap Minn). 2014;20(2 Cerebrovascular Disease):296-308.

16. Sur NB, Kozberg M, Desvigne-Nickens P, Silversides C, Bushnell C, Goldstein LB, et al. Improving stroke risk factor management focusing on health disparities and knowledge gaps. Stroke. 2024;55(1):248-58.
17. Massgeneralbrigham.org. (2024). Foods that help prevent stroke. [online] Available from https://www.massgeneralbrigham.org/en/about/newsroom/articles/foods-that-help-prevent-stroke. [Last accessed August, 2024]
18. Gallanagh S, Quinn TJ, Alexander J, Walters MR. Physical activity in the prevention and treatment of stroke. ISRN Neurol. 2011;2011:1-10.
19. Stroke Foundation - Australia. Quit smoking. [online] Available from https://strokefoundation.org.au/about-stroke/prevent-stroke/smoking. [Last accessed August, 2024]
20. Muschealth.org. Drinking & stroke risk. [online] Available from https://muschealth.org/medical-services/geriatrics-and-aging/healthy-aging/drinking-and-stroke-risk. [Last accessed August, 2024]
21. Heart.org. How High Blood Pressure can Lead to Stroke. [online] Available from https://www.heart.org/en/health-topics/high-blood-pressure/health-threats-from-high-blood-pressure/how-high-blood-pressure-can-lead-to-stroke. [Last accessed August, 2024]
22. Menet R, Bernard M, ElAli A. Hyperlipidemia in stroke pathobiology and therapy: Insights and perspectives. Front Physiol. 2018;9:488.
23. Akhtar N, Singh R, Kamran S, Joseph S, Morgan D, Uy RT, et al. Association between serum triglycerides and stroke type, severity, and prognosis. Analysis in 6558 patients. BMC Neurol. 2024;24(1):88.
24. Stroke.org. Diabetes and Stroke Prevention. [online] Available from https://www.stroke.org/en/about-stroke/stroke-risk-factors/diabetes-and-stroke-prevention. [Last accessed August, 2024]
25. Quiñones-Ossa GA, Lobo C, Garcia-Ballestas E, Florez WA, Moscote-Salazar LR, Agrawal A. Obesity and stroke: Does the paradox apply for stroke? Neurointervention. 2021;16(1):9-19.
26. Happiest Health. (2023). The sleeping epidemic: Decoding the link between OSA and strokes. [online] Available from https://www.happiesthealth.com/articles/sleep/link-between-osa-and-strokes. [Last accessed August, 2024]
27. Bos MJ, Koudstaal PJ, Hofman A, Ikram MA. Modifiable etiological factors and the burden of stroke from the Rotterdam study: A population-based cohort study. PLoS Med. 2014;11(4):e1001634.
28. Medscape.com. (2024). Stroke prevention. [online] Available from https://emedicine.medscape.com/article/323662-overview?form=fpf. [Last accessed August, 2024]
29. Wang Y, Meng R, Liu G, Cao C, Chen F, Jin K, et al. Intracranial atherosclerotic disease. Neurobiol Dis. 2019;124:118-32.
30. Zhu Z, Yu W. Update in the treatment of extracranial atherosclerotic disease for stroke prevention. Stroke Vasc Neurol. 2020;5(1):65-70.
31. Hopkinsmedicine.org. (2021). Moyamoya disease. [online] Available from https://www.hopkinsmedicine.org/health/conditions-and-diseases/moyamoya-disease. [Last accessed August, 2024]
32. Mok V, Kim JS. Prevention and management of cerebral small vessel disease. J Stroke. 2015;17(2):111.
33. Pillai AA, Tadi P, Kanmanthareddy A. (2023). Cardioembolic Stroke. [online] Available from https://www.ncbi.nlm.nih.gov/books/NBK536990/. [Last accessed August, 2024]
34. Goodfriend SD, Tadi P, Koury R. (2022). Carotid Artery Dissection. [online] Available from https://www.ncbi.nlm.nih.gov/books/NBK430835/. [Last accessed August, 2024]
35. Britt TB, Agarwal S. (2023). Vertebral Artery Dissection. [online] Available from https://www.ncbi.nlm.nih.gov/books/NBK441827/#:~:text=Vertebral%20artery%20dissection%20can%20be,carry%20a%20much%20worse%20prognosis. [Last accessed August, 2024]
36. Levine SR. Hypercoagulable states and stroke: A selective review. CNS Spectr. 2005;10(7):567-78.
37. Ford B, Peela S, Roberts C. Secondary prevention of ischemic stroke: Updated guidelines from AHA/ASA. Am Fam Physician. 2022;105(1):99-102.
38. Gannon K. Stroke systems of care: Dela J Public Health. 2023;9(3):16-9.
39. Salinas J, Schwamm LH. Behavioral interventions for stroke prevention: The need for a new conceptual model. Stroke. 2017;48(6):1706-14.
40. Towfighi A, Ovbiagele B. Health Equity and Actionable Disparities in stroke: 2022 update. Stroke. 2023;54(2):374-8.

CHAPTER 11

Recent Advances in Imaging of Acute Ischemic Stroke

Aneesh Mohimen

ABSTRACT

The use of advanced imaging techniques in acute ischemic stroke (AIS) has significantly improved patient outcomes, with studies like MR CLEAN (A randomized trial of intra-arterial treatment for acute ischemic stroke), ESCAPE (Randomized assessment of rapid endovascular treatment of ischemic stroke), and EXTEND IA (Endovascular therapy for ischemic stroke with perfusion-imaging selection) reshaping clinical protocols. However, in India, the integration of these techniques faces challenges due to limited accessibility, healthcare infrastructure disparities, and technology distribution. Achieving simple, uniform imaging protocols and evaluation criteria is crucial for clinical decision-making.

Keywords: AIS, Protocols, India, Technology.

INTRODUCTION

Over the past decade, the landscape of imaging in acute ischemic stroke (AIS) has undergone a transformative evolution, driven by groundbreaking findings from several pivotal randomized controlled trials. Studies such as MR CLEAN (A randomized trial of intra-arterial treatment for acute ischemic stroke),[1] ESCAPE (Randomized assessment of rapid endovascular treatment of ischemic stroke),[2] and EXTEND IA (Endovascular therapy for ischemic stroke with perfusion-imaging selection)[3] have not only reshaped clinical protocols but also emphasized the critical role of advanced imaging techniques in enhancing patient outcomes. These trials have collectively established endovascular therapy in the form of mechanical thrombectomy (MT), guided by precise imaging, as a standard of care, significantly extending the therapeutic window for ischemic stroke interventions.

In India, however, the integration of these advanced imaging modalities into routine clinical practice faces unique challenges. Despite the proven efficacy of modern imaging techniques, the accessibility of such services remains limited, particularly in rural and underserved areas. The disparity in healthcare infrastructure and the uneven distribution of technology exacerbate the gap between urban centers and less developed regions. There is a need for simple and uniform imaging protocols and evaluation criteria, for clinical decision making which can be widely applied and generalizable. The aim of this chapter is to briefly recount the bedrocks of acute stroke imaging and look at the emerging evidence leading to newer imaging paradigms.

PRINCIPLES AND TECHNIQUES OF IMAGING IN ACUTE ISCHEMIC STROKE

Imaging plays a pivotal role in the acute management of ischemic stroke, particularly through the evaluation of the three critical aspects—parenchyma, penumbra, and pipes. This tripartite approach helps clinicians assess the extent of the stroke, identify salvageable brain tissue, and decide on the most appropriate intervention. The basic premise of AIS imaging is simple enough: Assess the parenchyma to delineate the ischemic issue and rule out a hemorrhage, assess the intra- and extracranial vessels to detect the culprit occlusion and to plan MT, and finally quantify the salvageable for the unsalvageable brain tissue for patient selection for revascularization as well as prognostication.[4]

The bedrocks of the imaging modalities are CT scan and MRI (with their multiple protocols) based upon individual clinical scenarios. Digital subtraction angiography (DSA) has been completely supplanted as a purely diagnostic tool in view of excellent noninvasive vascular imaging techniques and is now used only when MT is planned based upon the clinical and noninvasive imaging parameters. The imaging techniques and protocols will not be new to anyone working in the field of neurosciences for any length of time; however, it is always prudent to review the same in a sequential manner, even if at the very least, it serves merely as a refresher for the experienced or an initial guide for the uninitiated. In the subsequent section, we will quickly refresh the well-established imaging paradigms and briefly consider the pros and cons of each. Rather than classifying the discussion based on modalities, we shall discuss subdivide the same based upon the pathological area of imaging for a more scientific approach to the topic. **Figure 1** shows the goals of imaging in AIS with a background of essential background clinical information.

IMAGING OF BRAIN PARENCHYMA

Imaging of the brain parenchyma primarily involves the use of CT and MRI scans to detect ischemic changes and exclude intracranial hemorrhage. Additionally parenchymal imaging serves to exclude stroke from stroke mimics like neoplasms, infections, demyelination, etc.

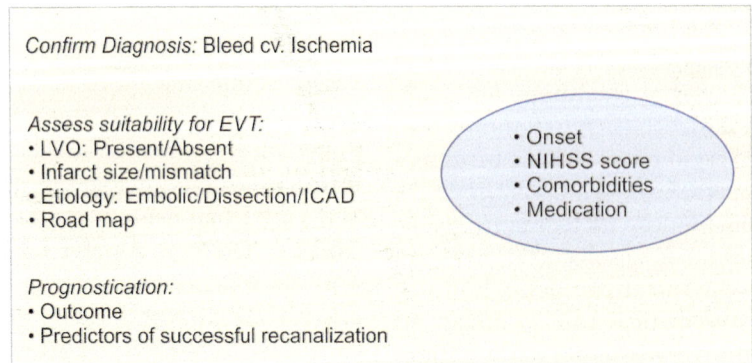

FIG. 1: Goals of imaging in AIS. Blue circle represents essential clinical information prior to starting imaging.
(AIS: acute ischemic stroke; EVT: endovascular treatment; ICAD: intracranial atherosclerotic disease; LVO: large vessel occlusion)

Noncontrast computed tomography (NCCT) is often the first-line imaging modality in the evaluation of suspected AIS due to its widespread availability, rapid acquisition time, and effectiveness in identifying early signs of ischemia and vascular occlusions. The first role of NCCT which can never be overemphasized is the exclusion of intracranial hemorrhage. This role has never changed over the decades since CT scan became the cornerstone of neurovascular imaging. NCCT is pivotal in detecting early signs of cerebral ischemia, which include loss of gray–white matter differentiation, hypoattenuation of brain tissue, and sulcal effacement.[5] These changes are often subtle initially but progress rapidly. Evaluation of the NCCT images in conventional and modified window settings is key to identifying hyperacute ischemic changes. Another significant finding on NCCT is the hyperdense artery sign, indicative of a clot in a blood vessel, typically seen as a bright white appearance on the scan within a cerebral artery, most commonly the middle cerebral artery (dense MCA/MCA dot/dense basilar sign). The same is a pointer toward an erythrocyte-rich thrombus which is useful in prognosticating the outcome of an endovascular procedure[6] and will be discussed later in the chapter. A point to be added in this section for young practitioners is the absolutely essential viewing of NCCT images in stroke window for better delineation of early ischemic changes **(Fig. 2)**.

ASPECTS: The Alberta Stroke Program Early CT Score (ASPECTS) is a 10-point quantitative score used to assess the extent of ischemic changes in the middle cerebral artery territory on NCCT.[4] It is designed to standardize the interpretation of CT findings and assist in clinical decision-making.

Posterior circulation ASPECTS (pc-ASPECTS): Similar to ASPECTS, the pc-ASPECTS is applied to the brainstem and cerebellum to assess ischemic changes within the posterior circulation. It scores from 10 (no ischemia) to 0 (extensive ischemia), covering specific brain regions including the thalamus, brainstem, and cerebellar hemispheres. In spite of widespread use, ASPECTS suffers from issues of inter-user variability and low sensitivity. The early trials[1] on endovascular revascularization used NCCT ASPECTS of 6 or more as a selection criteria for MT **(Fig. 3)**.

Magnetic resonance imaging is a powerful tool in the diagnosis and management of AIS, offering detailed insights into brain tissue integrity, perfusion, and the extent of ischemic damage. While CT is often the first-line imaging modality due to its availability

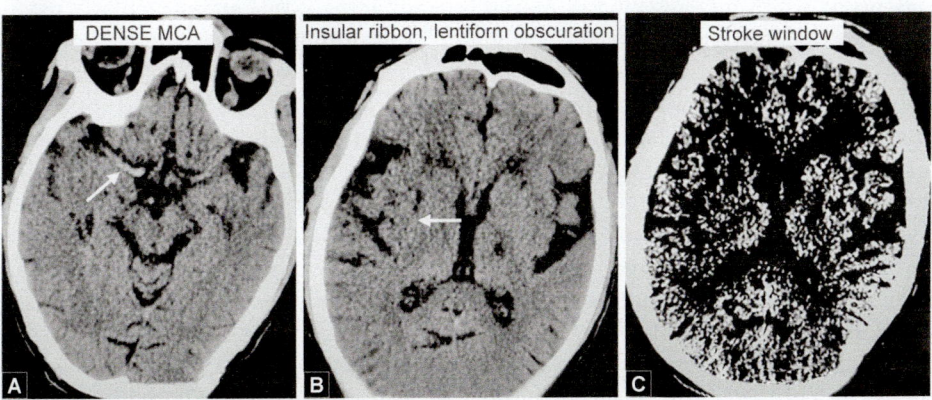

FIGS. 2A TO C: Early ischemic changes on NCCT.
(NCCT: noncontrast computed tomography)

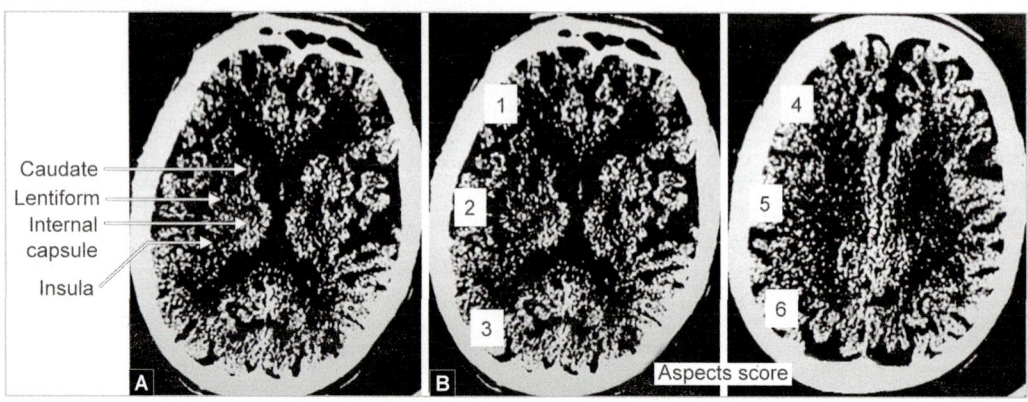

FIGS. 3A AND B: The Alberta Stroke Program Early CT Score (ASPECTS) on NCCT.
(NCCT: noncontrast computed tomography)

and speed, MRI has specific advantages that make it indispensable in certain clinical scenarios. This section explores the situations where MRI outperforms CT, the protocols used in MRI for stroke assessment, and the utility of MR perfusion techniques in AIS. MRI is particularly valuable in AIS when detailed tissue characterization is required, especially in the following scenarios:[7,8]

- *Early detection of ischemic stroke*: Diffusion-weighted imaging (DWI), a core MRI sequence, is highly sensitive to early ischemic changes. DWI can detect ischemic lesions within minutes of stroke onset, long before they are visible on CT.[9] This makes MRI the preferred modality in patients who present early after symptom onset or when the time of onset is unclear.
- *Identification of small or lacunar strokes*: MRI is superior to CT in identifying small infarcts, particularly in the brainstem or other regions where small vessel disease predominates.
- *Assessment of stroke mimics*: MRI is invaluable in differentiating ischemic stroke from stroke mimics such as seizures, migraines, or demyelinating diseases. Sequences like fluid-attenuated inversion recovery (FLAIR) and DWI provide detailed tissue contrast, helping clinicians distinguish between these conditions.
- *Evaluation of posterior fossa strokes*: CT often has limitations in visualizing the posterior fossa due to beam-hardening artifacts from the skull base. MRI, however, provides clear imaging of the cerebellum, brainstem, and other posterior fossa structures, making it the preferred modality for detecting strokes in these areas.
- *Assessment of hemorrhagic transformation*: MRI is more sensitive than CT in detecting small hemorrhages that can occur as a complication of ischemic stroke or as part of hemorrhagic transformation after thrombolysis. Gradient echo (GRE) sequences or susceptibility-weighted imaging (SWI) are particularly useful for this purpose.

In summary, while CT is faster and more widely available, MRI offers superior sensitivity and specificity in various scenarios, making it a crucial tool in the comprehensive assessment of AIS. A comprehensive MRI protocol for AIS typically includes several key sequences, each providing unique information about the brain's status. The following are the most commonly used MRI sequences in stroke imaging **(Figs. 4 and 5)**:

- *Diffusion-weighted imaging (DWI)*: DWI is the cornerstone of stroke imaging with MRI. It detects cytotoxic edema, which

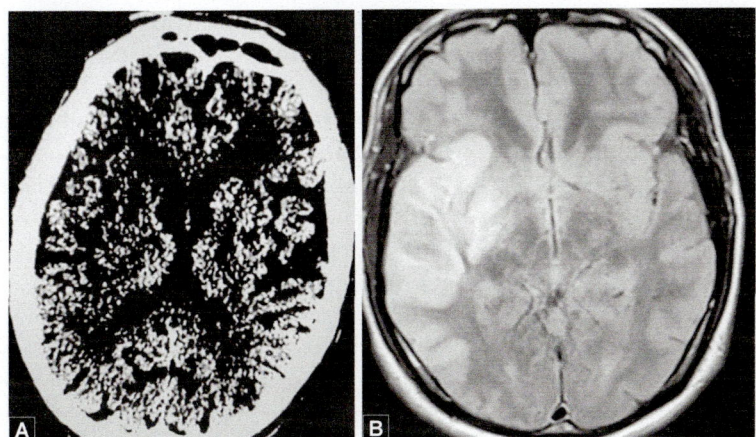

FIGS. 4A AND B: NCCT (stroke window) versus MRI (FLAIR) in detecting the ischemic neuroparenchyma in a case of right MCA territory stroke.
(FLAIR: fluid-attenuated inversion recovery; MCA: middle cerebral artery; NCCT: noncontrast computed tomography)

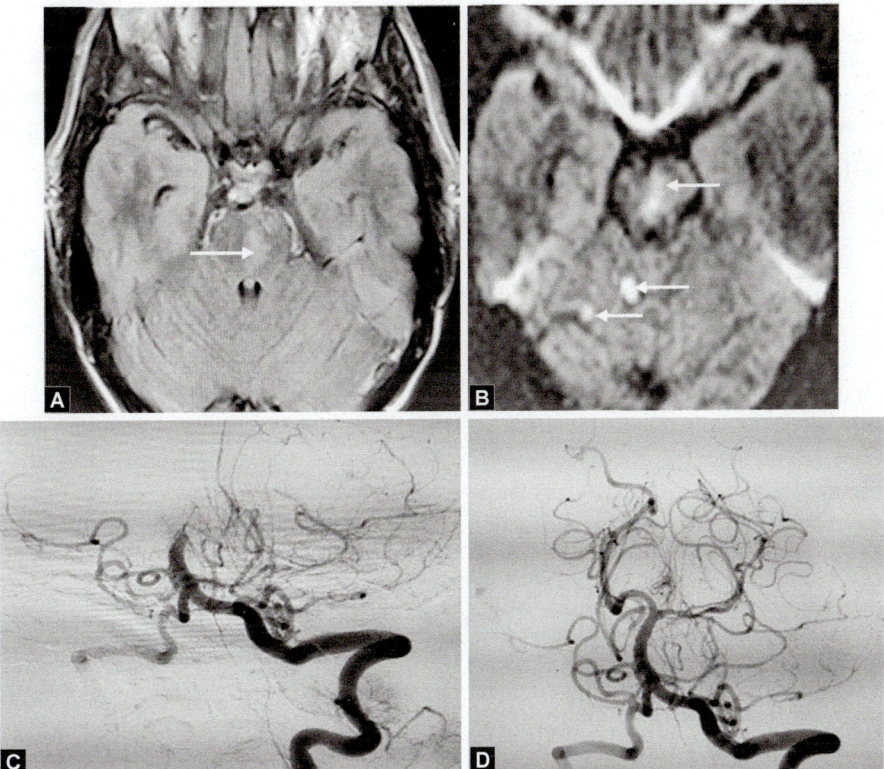

FIGS. 5A TO D: Role of MRI in posterior circulation stroke. (A) FLAIR axial showing acute pontine infarct; and (B) DWI showing additional infarcts in the right cerebellar hemisphere in a case of acute basilar artery occlusion, pre (C) and post (D) mechanical thrombectomy.
(DWI: diffusion-weighted imaging; FLAIR: fluid-attenuated inversion recovery)

occurs early in ischemic stroke, allowing for the identification of the ischemic core. The high sensitivity of DWI makes it the sequence of choice for diagnosing acute strokes, often showing changes within minutes of stroke onset.

- *Fluid-attenuated inversion recovery (FLAIR)*: In the context of stroke, FLAIR can help identify lesions older than 4.5 hours, which is particularly useful when the exact time of stroke onset is unknown. A mismatch between DWI and FLAIR can indicate a hyperacute stroke and guide thrombolytic therapy decisions.
- *Gradient echo (GRE) or susceptibility-weighted imaging (SWI)*: These sequences are highly sensitive to blood products and are used to detect hemorrhages, including microbleeds, which may not be visible on CT. This is crucial in assessing patients for hemorrhagic transformation or in determining eligibility for thrombolysis.

IMAGING OF INTRA- AND EXTRACRANIAL VESSELS (PIPES)

The assessment of "pipes", or the vascular architecture, involves the use of angiography techniques, including CT angiography (CTA), and MR angiography (MRA). These imaging techniques are vital for visualizing occlusions and stenoses in the cerebral arteries. Identifying the location and extent of arterial blockages enables clinicians to determine the feasibility and approach for revascularization procedures.[10-12] It is beyond the purview of this chapter to explore in detail the physical principles and all technical aspects of each of these individual modalities; however, in the general chapter of stroke imaging, it is prudent to include the undermentioned points with regard to noninvasive vascular imaging in cases of AIS.

Computed tomography angiogram is the most robust technique with least motion related limitations because of its short duration of acquisition. Additionally, it is the best method for demonstrating calcium in the vessel wall or in a plaque.[4] The natural limitations of CT scan are radiation exposure,[13] which is probably moot in a case of AIS and the theoretical risk of nephrotoxicity due to iodinated contrast. The introduction of multiphase CT angiogram for assessment of collaterals, which shall be discussed later in this chapter, is an additional benefit of CT over MRI for neurovascular imaging. Isotropic image reconstruction of the new-generation CT scan machines now permits excellent depiction of even median vessel occlusions which imperative in the progressively expanding indication of MT in MVO.

Magnetic resonance angiographic techniques can broadly be divided into those which require exogenous contrast [CE MRA (contrast enhanced MR angiogram)] as opposed to techniques which generate endogenous contrast based upon blood flow such as Time-of-Flight (TOF) angiography.[14] The 2019 update to the 2018 stroke recommendations permit both CT and MR angiogram for evaluation of cerebral vasculature. It has, therefore, largely become an institutional protocol as to which method is employed. Whatever be the technique of choice, it is essential that the vascular imaging commences from the aortic arch and be carried out to the top of the cranial vault. This will give a proper road map for the interventionist in planning a MT and also delineate the extracranial vessels which may be a source of thrombus, or provide significant challenges in negotiating endovascular hardware to their site of intracranial occlusions. Attempts at MT without proper evaluation of the aortic arch, cervical and intracranial vasculature on noninvasive vascular imaging may at times end up in disastrous results further complicating the condition of the patient **(Figs. 6 to 8)**.[15]

CHAPTER 11: Recent Advances in Imaging of Acute Ischemic Stroke

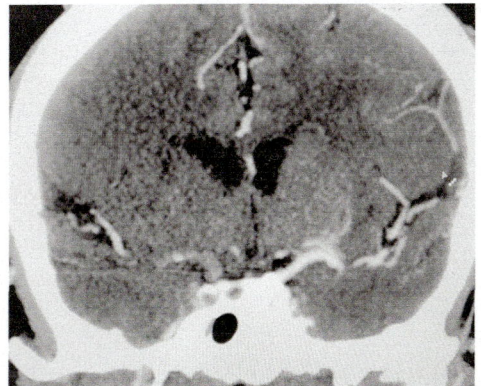

FIG. 6: Right ICA terminus and proximal MCA (M1) occlusion on CTA.
(CTA: CT angiography; ICA: internal carotid artery; MCA: middle cerebral artery)

IMAGING OF COLLATERALS

The evolution of advanced neuroimaging has increased understanding of cerebrovascular hemodynamic and the progression of healthy brain tissue from ischemic to infarct. This newer understanding helps in a better patient selection for reperfusion, especially in the era of ever widening indications for the same. The protocols are now shifting from a "time" to "tissue" based approach. The "Time is brain" concept is progressively evolving into the "Collateral Clock" concept. In view of the same, assessment of the collateral brain circulation plays a vital role in evaluating potentially viable brain tissue. Collaterals

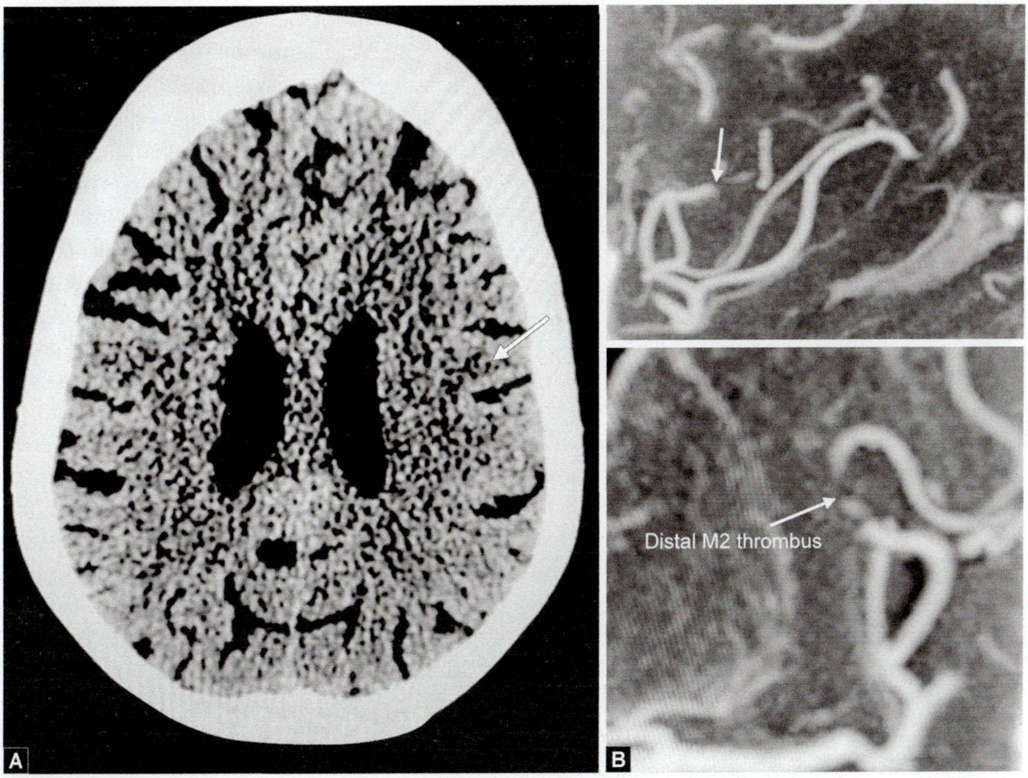

FIGS. 7A AND B: NCCT showing small left precentral gyrus infarct with CTA depicting a distal left M2 segment MCA thrombus.
(CTA: CT angiography; MCA: middle cerebral artery; NCCT: noncontrast computed tomography)

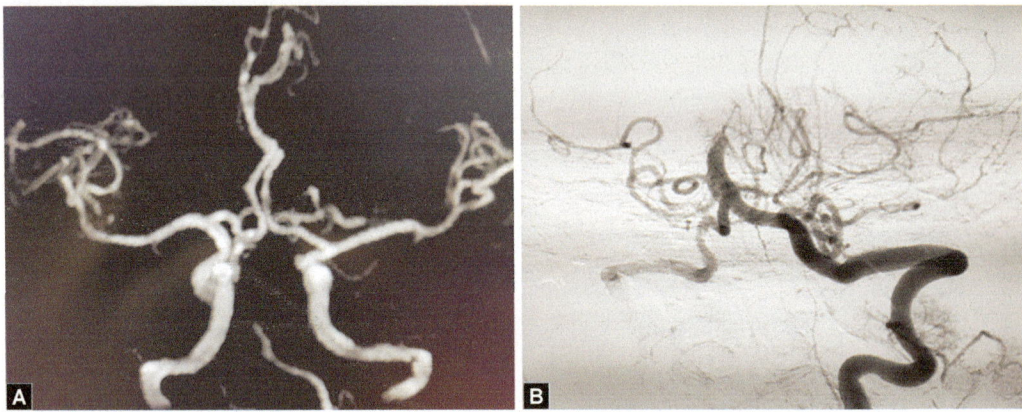

FIGS. 8A AND B: TOF MRA and DSA showing a midbasilar artery occlusion in a case of posterior circulation stroke.
(DSA: digital subtraction angiography; MRA: MR angiography; TOF: time-of-flight)

TABLE 1: Cerebral collateral circulation.

Structural classification	Functional classification
Circle of Willis (proximal large collaterals)	Primary
Microvascular intracranial: • Leptomeningeal (pial) • Subcortical	Secondary
Extracranial	Tertiary

can broadly be classified based upon a structural or functional approach as depicted in **Table 1**.[16]

The full anatomy and pathophysiology are elucidated eloquently in a number of excellent review articles. For the purpose of this chapter, we will focus only upon the imaging of collaterals and the clinical implications of the same. The unparalleled temporal resolution of DSA makes it the best modality for assessing cerebral hemodynamic; however, it is impractical to perform a DSA in all patients with stroke merely for the purpose of assessing collaterals. The technological boon in this regard has been evolution of CT scan technology and the development of newer generation multidetector CT scan machines which have rapid tube rotation times leading to quicker brain coverage and, therefore, multiple coverages over a single contrast circulation time. Once neurovascular imaging (primarily with CTA) became mandatory in the evaluation of acute stroke following the MR CLEAN trial,[1] protocols rapidly evolved into the development of multiphase CT angiography (MP-CTA) for assessment of collaterals along with vessel occlusion. Multiple different collateral scores have been propounded, based on either single phase or multiphase acquisition. A summary of various single-phase collateral scoring methods is presented in **Table 2**.[17-22]

The technique of MP-CTA described by Menon et al. involves the acquisition of images at multiple time points during a single contrast injection.[17] Typically, this includes at least three phases: arterial, venous, and delayed. Each phase provides valuable information about the timing and extent of blood flow through the cerebral arteries and veins, offering insights into the dynamics of cerebral perfusion that are not possible with traditional single-phase CTA. It is essential

TABLE 2: Various collateral scoring methods on single phase/arterial phase of CTA.[17]

Scoring method	Description
American Society of Interventional and Therapeutic Neuroradiology/Society of Interventional Radiology (ASITN/SIR)[18]	Grades 0-4, based on the extent of collateral vessels filling the ischemic territory compared to the contralateral hemisphere
Tan collateral score[19]	Evaluates collaterals at the clot location using a 10-point scale, where higher scores indicate better collateral status
Regional leptomeningeal collateral score[20]	Assesses collaterals on a regional basis in the middle cerebral artery territory, scoring from 0 (no collaterals) to 3 (exuberant collaterals)
Maas collateral score[21]	Quantifies collaterals based on their prominence compared to the primary arterial occlusion, with scores indicating poor to good collateral flow
Capillary index score[22]	Assesses the presence of capillary blush in the ischemic territory, used primarily to assess the viability of tissue and guide revascularization decisions

(CTA: computed tomography angiography)

TABLE 3: MP-CTA collateral status with pathological correlate.

MP-CTA collateral status	Pathological correlate
Minimal/no collaterals	Irreversible damage
• Single phase delay • Impaired washout in 3rd phase: Severely ischemic brain	• Severely ischemic brain • Potentially salvageable with quick reperfusion
• One phase delay • Washout in 3rd phase	Mildly ischemic brain

(MP-CTA: multiphase computed tomography angiography)

that the first (early arterial) phase covers the vasculature from the aortic arch to the top of the vault while the other two phases are skull-base to vault scans, each with a delay of 4 s. The pathological correlates of the MP-CTA scores are detailed in **Table 3**.

■ PERFUSION IMAGING IN ACUTE ISCHEMIC STROKE

Perfusion imaging is the physiological sibling to the anatomical information gleaned on collateral imaging. Recent perfusion techniques whether they be CT or MRI based give a relatively accurate interpretation of tissue circulation and an inference of the metabolic milieu resulting out of ischemia.

We shall now take a brief look into the technical aspects of CT and MRI perfusion followed by a dive into the evidences of perfusion-based imaging related to decision making in AIS.

Computed Tomography Perfusion in Acute Ischemic Stroke

Computed tomography perfusion (CTP) imaging is an advanced diagnostic tool that plays a crucial role in the management of AIS, offering detailed insights into the cerebral blood flow dynamics at the tissue level.[23] This section outlines the timing, protocols, and key parameters of CTP that are instrumental in clinical decision-making **(Tables 4 and 5)**.

TABLE 4: Normal values of CT perfusion parameters.

CBV	4–5 mL/100 g
CBF	• GM: 80 mL/100 g/min • WM: 20 mL/100 g/min
MTT	4–5 s
T_{max}	<6 s

(CBF: cerebral blood flow; CBV: cerebral blood volume; MTT: mean transit time)

TABLE 5: Quantification of infarct core and penumbra (as per DAWN and DEFUSE 3 trials).

Infarct core	Penumbra
CBV < 2 mL/100 g	MTT > 145% (as compared to normal side)
CBF: 30–45% (as compared to normal side)	T_{max} > 6 s

(CBF: cerebral blood flow; CBV: cerebral blood volume; MTT: mean transit time)

- *Protocol of CT perfusion*: The timing of CTP is critical, ideally performed immediately after noncontrast CT and before CT angiography. The technical essentials for an ideal CTP are injection of contrast into a large vein (ideally the antecubital vein) and at least a eight cm longitudinal coverage of the head during the perfusion scan.
- *Parameters for clinical decision making*:
  - *Cerebral blood flow (CBF)*: Measures the volume of blood passing through a given amount of brain tissue per unit time. A significant reduction in CBF is indicative of the ischemic core.
  - *Cerebral blood volume (CBV)*: Reflects the amount of blood in a given brain volume at a particular time. Decreases in CBV suggest irreversible brain tissue damage.
  - *Mean transit time (MTT)*: Represents the average time it takes for blood to pass through a segment of brain tissue. Prolongation of MTT often correlates with tissue at risk but potentially salvageable if perfusion is restored.
  - T_{max}, *or time to maximum of the residue function*, is a critical parameter which quantifies the delay in blood flow to brain tissue and is instrumental in identifying areas of the brain that are ischemic but potentially salvageable (penumbra). A prolonged T_{max} indicates delayed cerebral blood flow, which may still be reversible with appropriate intervention. Clinically, a T_{max} delay of >6 seconds is commonly used to delineate the ischemic penumbra from infarcted tissue.

Magnetic Resonance Perfusion in Acute Ischemic Stroke

Two techniques are used, based upon exogenous or endogenous contrast. A third MR perfusion technique called dynamic contrast-enhanced perfusion (DCE perfusion) does not have much clinical applicability in AIS **(Fig. 9)**.[4,24]

- *Dynamic susceptibility contrast (DSC) perfusion*: DSC is the most widely used MR perfusion technique in stroke imaging. It involves the injection of a gadolinium-based contrast agent and the rapid acquisition of images to measure changes in signal intensity as the contrast passes through the brain. This technique also provides information about cerebral blood flow (CBF), cerebral blood volume (CBV), and mean transit time (MTT). As opposed to CTP, DSC perfusion only gives a relative nonquantitative idea of tissue perfusion and hence the parameters are all prefixed by the alphabet "r" indicating the relativeness.
- *Arterial spin labeling (ASL)*: ASL is a noncontrast MR perfusion technique that

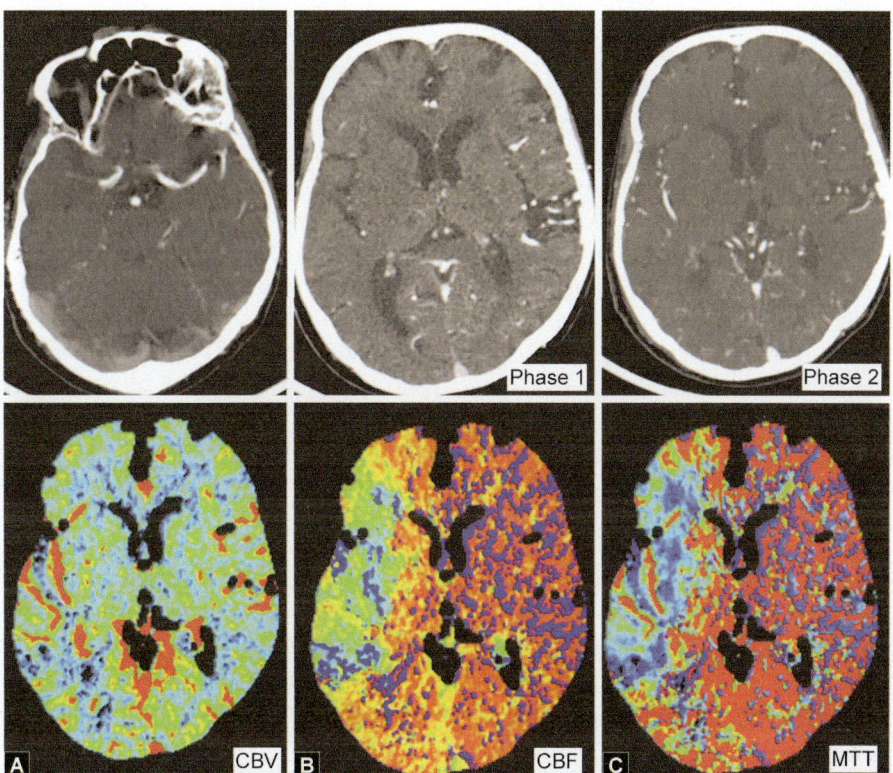

FIGS. 9A TO C: Three phase CTA and CTP in a case of right MCA occlusion demonstrating poor collateral score (two phase delay) and minimal mismatch suggestive of irreversible damage in the involved right MCA territory.

(CBF: cerebral blood flow; CBV: cerebral blood volume; MTT: mean transit time; MCA: middle cerebral artery)

uses magnetically labeled arterial blood as an endogenous tracer to measure cerebral perfusion. ASL provides quantitative measurements of CBF and is effective in detecting areas of hypoperfusion.

IMAGING FOR VIABLE PARENCHYMA—WHERE ARE WE NOW?

Both collateral imaging and perfusion imaging are theoretically excellent and robust methods to demonstrate the difference between viable and nonviable parenchyma in the setting of acute ischemia. However, both methods come with their own inherent set of disadvantages because of which a single gold standard has so far being difficult to home upon. Perfusion techniques are exquisitely sensitive to patient motion and even a slight head movement during scan acquisition can render the study uninterpretable. Quantitative perfusion-based selective criteria used in the different trials are difficult to replicate in day-to-day clinical work either due to the absence volumetric software or lack of time and expertise. Often, due to paucity of time, perfusion maps are qualitatively interpreted for clinical decision making. While the same usually suffices, there may be cases in which data is misinterpreted reading of an incorrect decision to regarding revascularization.

Collateral imaging on CT angiography especially MP-CTA is nongeneralizable due to the wide variety of CT scan machines. The collateral score is dependent upon the scan times which are in turn a property of the CT machine tube rotation time. The latter varies depending upon the generation and type of CT scanner and hence collateral scores obtained in different machines may give different interpretations. Furthermore, the wide variety of different collateral scores and single phase or multiphase protocols have so far not been homogenized into a single recommendation. For instance, in spite of the MP-CTA collateral score theoretically being a better technique than the single-phase method, the recent MR CLEAN LATE trial[25] used a single-phase collateral score in its protocol. While the definite reason for this has not been mentioned, it is probably due to different protocols in different study centers.

With this background on the imaging in AIS, **Table 6**[26] highlights the different imaging paradigms and protocols used by the major trials over the past decade. It is prudent we consider these before we progress the recent trials and the imaging protocols used in the search for widening of indications for MT.

ACUTE STROKE IMAGING RECOMMENDATIONS: 2019 UPDATE TO 2018 AHA/ASA GUIDELINES[27]

The American Heart Association/American Stroke Association (AHA/ASA) published the 2018 guidelines to the management of AIS which were subsequently updated in 2019 (which have subsequently not been updated or revised). These guidelines were published in the wake of the DAWN and DEFUSE 3 trials which left no ambiguity in the benefit of extended window MT if certain imaging selection parameters were met. **Table 7** summarizes the different imaging protocols with their levels of evidence in the 2019 update used for patient selection for revascularization. **Table 8** details the delayed window period imaging inclusion criteria for revascularization used in the DAWN and DEFUSE 3 trials, respectively **(Fig. 10)**.

Directions of Research after 2019

By the end of the second decade of the millennium, the treatment of AIS had been revolutionized as compared to the evidence at the end of the first decade. The first half overwhelmingly confirmed the benefit of MT in patients with large vessel occlusion (LVO) proved on noninvasive imaging with hitherto unseen NNT figures. Subsequent research looked at extending the indications

TABLE 6: Different imaging protocols used in the major stroke trials over the last decade.

CT name	Imaging modality used	Primary imaging criteria
MR CLEAN[1]	CT, CT angiography	Vessel occlusion in anterior circulation
ESCAPE[2]	CT, CT angiography	Small infarct core, good collateral circulation
EXTEND IA[3]	CT, CT angiography, CT perfusion	Small infarct core, presence of salvageable penumbra
DEFUSE 3[24]	MRI, CT perfusion	Ischemic core ≤70 mL, mismatch between core and penumbra
DAWN[26]	CT, CT angiography, CT perfusion	Mismatch between clinical deficit and infarct volume

TABLE 7: Levels of evidence for imaging protocols as summarized in 2019 update to the 2018 guidelines.

Imaging recommendation	Level of evidence
NCCT to rule out hemorrhage before IVT	IA
MRI to rule hemorrhage before IVT	IB
CTA with CTP/MRA, DWI ± MR perfusion in select cases	IA
Time of onset unknown: FLAIR–DWI mismatch for selection of IVT	IIA
• Patient selection for MT in LVO—time of onset 6–24 hours • CTP or DWI ± MR perfusion (Only when patients meet eligibility criteria from DAWN/DEFUSE 3 trial)	IA

(DWI: diffusion-weighted imaging; FLAIR: fluid-attenuated inversion recovery; IVT: intravenous thrombolysis; NCCT: noncontrast computed tomography)

TABLE 8: Delayed window period inclusion criteria as per the DAWN and DEFUSE 3 trials.

Trial	Imaging inclusion criteria

DAWN[26]	• <1/3 MCA territory involved (CT/MRI)
	• Intracranial ICA/M1-MCA occlusion (CT/MRI)
	• Mismatch present (either of 3 definitions):
	  ○ >80 years age, NIHSS > 10, core volume < 21 mL
	  ○ <80 years age, NIHSS > 10, core volume < 31 mL
	  ○ <80 years age, NIHSS > 20, core volume < 51 mL

DEFUSE 3[24]	• ICA/M1-MCA occlusion
	• Mismatch on CTP/MRI:
	  ○ Ischemic core < 70 mL
	  ○ Mismatch ratio > 1.8
	  ○ Mismatch volume > 15 mL

(ICA: internal carotid artery; MCA: middle cerebral artery)

for MT as compared to the relatively stringent selection criteria of the landmark MR CLEAN trial.[25] While collaterals core and multiphase CTA had become widely established, easy to use, and with widespread acceptance in the imaging protocols, the same had still not made its way into the imaging recommendations. As previously mentioned, expansion of indications for MT was explored especially in the setting of large core. Furthermore, the parameters for perfusion-based selection criteria are not objective and need for simplification was felt justified. We shall be now discussing recent trial-based evidence in these contexts over the next section.

LARGE CORE INFARCTS

Since the publication of the 2019 update to the 2018 AHA/ASA recommendations,[27] newer research has focused on expanding the indications of revascularization in AIS. The prime target has been low ASPECTS strokes which had hitherto been stringently excluded. The salient results of a number of trials published in the last few years are detailed in **Table 9**.[28-32] While the purview of the chapter is not to cover selection for revascularization, it would be amiss not to mention these trials, if at the very least to highlight the different imaging paradigms used by each.

The slew of large core trials has overwhelmingly shown a significant benefit in morbidity in the endovascular therapy (EVT) arm of large core LVO strokes (ASPECTS < 5). The LASTE[32] and TENSION[30] trials have been the only ones to show mortality benefit in large core infarct patient

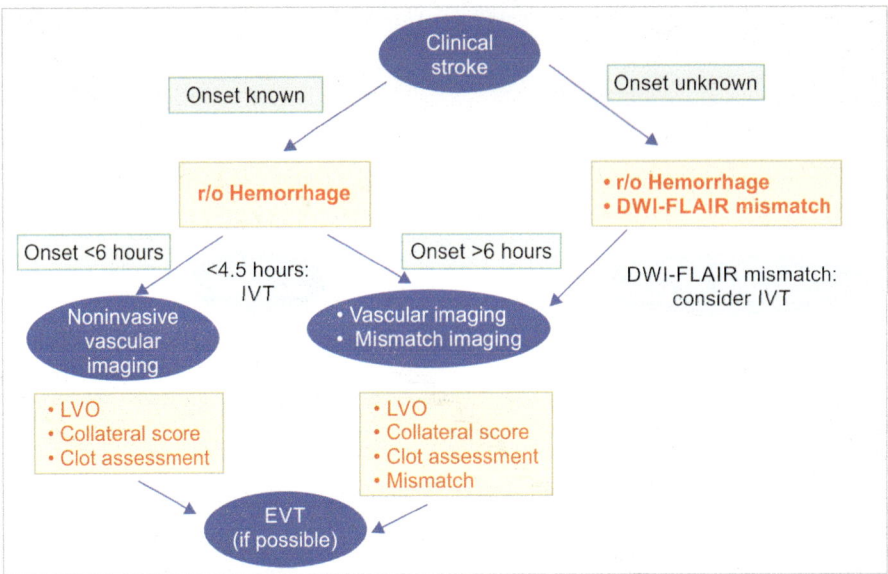

FIG. 10: Algorithm for revascularization in acute ischemic stroke based upon the 2019 update to the 2018 recommendations of the AHA/ASA guidelines.[27]
(AHA/ASA: American Heart Association/American Stroke Association; DWI: diffusion-weighted imaging; FLAIR: fluid-attenuated inversion recovery; IVT: intravenous thrombolysis; EVT: endovascular therapy; LVO: large vessel occlusion)

TABLE 9: Salient results of trials on mechanical thrombectomy (MT) in low ASPECTS strokes.

Name of trial	Number of patients	Selection criteria	Salient results
SELECT2[28] (Randomized controlled trial to optimize patient's selection for endovascular treatment in AIS)	352 patients (31 centers)	ASPECTS 3–5 Or CTP core > 50 mL	• mRS 0–2 • EVT arm: 20% • Medical Management • Arm: 7% • *Stopped early*
ANGEL-ASPECT[29] (Endovascular therapy in acute anterior circulation large vessel occlusive patients with a large infarct core)	456 patients (46 centers)	ASPECTS 3–5 Or ASPECTS 0–2 with CTP core 70–100 mL	• Functional independence at 90 day • EVT: 30% • Medical management: 12% • SICH in EVT arm: 6.1%
TENSION[30] (Efficacy and safety of thrombectomy in stroke with extended lesion and extended time window)	253 patients (40 centers)	ASPECTS 3–5 on NCCT	• Efficacy after EVT associated with shift in mRS toward better outcome at 90 days [odds ratio (OR) 2.58 (95% CI 1.60–4.15); *p* = 0.0001] • SICH: EVT—6% • Medical management: 5% • Mean mRS (EVT)—4%

Continued

Continued

Name of trial	Number of patients	Selection criteria	Salient results
TESLA[31] (Thrombectomy for emergent salvage of large anterior circulation ischemic stroke)	300 patients	NCCT only Anterior circulation LVO ASPECTS: 2–5	• mRS 0–2 at 90 days insignificant (trend toward benefit in EVT arm) • mRS 0–3 vs. 4–6 (significant) • 30% in EVT arm • 20% medical management arm • EVT mortality: 35% • SICH (EVT): 4%
LASTE[32] (Large stroke therapy evaluation)	324 patients	ASPECTS: 0–5 (predominantly MRI)	• Increased odds of good outcome in EVT compared with medical management [OR, 1.63 (95% CI 1.29–2.06); $p < 0.0001$] • NNT: 4.2 • SICH: Close to 10% in EVT arm

(ASPECTS: Alberta Stroke Program Early Computed Tomography Score; EVT: endovascular therapy; NCCT: noncontrast computed tomography; SICH: symptomatic intracerebral hemorrhage)

undergoing EVT. However, the overall morbidity numbers expectedly remain low as compared to previous earlier RCTs which have predominantly included patients with ASPECTS > 5. The rates of symptomatic intracerebral hemorrhage (SICH) are also higher in the large core group (ranging from 4 to 10%). These results of these trials, while providing considerable encouragement for the previously considered "unsalvageable" low ASPECTS LVO group, bring different socioeconomic questions to the fore, especially in the Indian setting. It would require an extremely skilled counselor to explain the likelihood of a low benefit (good mRS < 40% and mortality > 30%) with a relatively costly procedure of EVT. Future studies in the Indian setting might provide insight into both the results, and the consent of families for performance of EVT in the group with uncertain benefit. While the trial results and a highly significant "*p* value" provide great hope to the medical professional, it may be difficult to convince the next of kin of a patient from a lower socioeconomic strata to consent for an EVT explaining that the chances of a "good outcome" are 3 in 10 as opposed to 2 in 10 if no procedure is done.

IMAGING PROTOCOLS: NEW EVIDENCE (MR CLEAN LATE TRIAL)

Patients with AIS due to anterior circulation LVO were selected based on the presence of collateral flow on CTA in the late window, and allocated to receive MT versus medical management only.[25] A total of 535 patients who were eligible for late-window EVT were randomly assigned to either EVT or medical management on the basis of the presence or absence of collateral flow on CT angiogram. The EVT group had a shift toward lower mRS

[OR 1.67 (95% CI 1.20–2.32)]. The patients in the endovascular arm had significantly better functional outcome at 90 days. While there were higher rates of SICH in this arm, the same was not significant and were similar to the rates of SICH noted in the DEFUSE 3 (24) and DAWN (26) trials. The overall outcome benefits were lesser than the DAWN and DEFUSE 3 trials, and the reason for the same was postulated as that of patients selected for MT based upon the DAWN and DEFUSE 3 criteria (already preexisting in The Netherlands national guidelines) were excluded from the MR CLEAN LATE trial.

The results of this trial may in the future lead to patient selection for delayed window revascularization be based purely upon collateral score rather than perfusion imaging. Incorporation of the results of these latest trials into guidelines is still awaited.

IMAGING BEYOND THE "P"S

While the holy grail of acute stroke imaging still remains timely patient selection for revascularization, the role of imaging and information gleaned from the same does not end here. There are a few areas where imaging provides vital information to the intrepid observer, which if incorporated into regular clinical practice will assist the interventionist and also be useful in prognostication and preprocedure counseling.

Thrombus Characterization in Acute Ischemic Stroke

Since the established benefit of MT in AIS, multiple studies have attempted to qualify thrombus character in a bid to prognosticate ease of MT. The ease of removal of RBC-rich thrombus versus fibrin-rich thrombus is well established. Preprocedure thrombus characterization would also help prognosticate the outcome, duration of procedure, and even decide on the need for conscious sedation versus full general anesthesia for MT. Thrombus characterization is largely divided into thrombus burden, location, and composition (i.e., RBC rich vs. fibrin rich).

Thrombus burden has been eyeballed over the past decade by the clot burden score which is easier and required less software constraints. Ji Hoe Heo et al.[33] have suggested that thrombus volume and length quantification on NCCT by pixel segmentation and automated calculation by software serve as a more accurate thrombus load predictor than clot burden score or software based calculations on CT angiography. Based upon appropriate thrombus characterization, at least three thrombus-based predictors of recanalization can be elucidated:

1. Thrombus length as opposed to thrombus burden is likely a more effective marker of difficult recanalization.
2. RBC-rich thrombus is easier to remove than of fibrin-rich thrombus.
3. Qualifying an occlusion as a definite thrombus as opposed to thrombus superimposed with underlying intracranial atherosclerosis.

Another parameter described to identify an erythrocyte-rich thrombus is presence of contrast permeability. An increase in 10 HU from baseline NCCT value of the thrombus on CTA source images has been described as a marker for the same.[34]

Predictors of Intracranial Atherosclerotic Stenosis on CT Angiogram

As with thrombus characterization and burden quantification, the advent of widespread MT has also necessitated the detection of intracranial atherosclerotic stenosis (ICAS) to prepare the interventionist prior to a thrombectomy procedure. Suspicion of ICAS prior to thrombectomy procedure will allow the interventionist to be ready with suitable hardware and also allow them to pre-empt complications and the duration of the procedure. ICAS (with or without an underlying thrombus) can create multiple problems during an MT procedure, namely vessel dissection and rupture, insufficient device expansion and device damage, vasospasm and inadvertent device detachment.

Some of the baseline imaging predictors for underlying ICAS are presence of calcium at the site of occlusion, smaller clot burden score, and a higher collateral score (due to a long standing ICAS).[35] Additionally, it is prudent to mention angiographic predictors of ICAS which may necessitate early conversion to intracranial stenting such as reocclusion and inadequate device deployment.

PREDICTORS OF HEMORRHAGIC TRANSFORMATION

Since the dawn of revascularization therapy for AIS, the critical limiting factor has always been the risk of intraparenchymal hemorrhage. As opposed to acute coronary thrombosis, reopening of acute occlusion of the cerebral vessels is associated with a definite increased risk of ICH due to reperfusion of brain nonviable tissue. Over the last decade, once class IA level of evidence for MT for AIS with LVO became established, subsequent research has been directed toward extending the indications for revascularization such as extending the window period and progressive inclusion of large core infarcts. It, therefore, is useful to attempt to prognosticate ICH while planning management of an AIS especially if revascularization is being considered.

The following imaging markers have been propounded as having an increased risk of ICH with different revascularization techniques.[36,37]

- *Intravenous thrombolysis (IVT)*:
  - Infarct size (>70–80 mL)
  - Clot length/density
  - Chronic small vessel ischemic disease (SVID)
  - Side
- *Endovascular therapy (EVT)*:
  - Collateral score
  - Proximal clot
  - Longer clot
  - Erythrocyte poor clot
  - Underlying ICAS

ARTIFICIAL INTELLIGENCE IN ACUTE ISCHEMIC STROKE MANAGEMENT

No discussion on medical imaging in the current era is complete without a discussion on artificial intelligence (AI). AI algorithms have rapidly integrated themselves into imaging research at the very least, if not yet into regular clinical practice. In the setting of AIS, AI-based research has sought to identify and predict different outcomes. A systematic review by Akay et al. in 2023[38] assessed publications and found three major groups of AI-based clinical decision support systems (CDSSs).

1. Extraction of stroke scores (not relevant to imaging)
2. AI models to identify patients for easier treatment selection
3. Models to predict future outcomes (including success of MT)

These models are more advanced from the automated software in existence for a few years, which have been used to essentially calculate ASPECTS (e-ASPECTS) and perfusion parameters. However, there is still an enormous heterogeneity in the AI models, selection of baseline data and validation studies. While promising in their concept, there appears to be some distance before AI makes its way into regular clinical practice. None of the major trials thus far have used AI models in patient selection or for prognostication.

CONCLUSION

The basic principles of imaging in AIS have remained the same over the past decade, as largely have the imaging modalities and protocols. The changing landscape has been in the progressively widening inclusion criteria for revascularization which is associated with different components of the imaging parameters as part of the selection. The question of CT versus MRI as the better modality still stands unsolved and is largely left at the mercy of institutional protocols. It had seemed 5 years back that perfusion imaging would be the cornerstone in selection of patients for delayed window thrombectomy; however, the results of recent trials with collateral imaging as selection criteria have suggested that may be the latter finds its way into the recommendations. In the Indian context, the protocols are still more diverse based upon individual and institutional preferences. Newer trials and guidelines may shed more light on the path toward the holy grail of "one common single imaging modality" for patient selection for revascularization in AIS, although that seems someway in the distance.

REFERENCES

1. Berkhemer OA, Fransen PS, Beumer D, van den Berg LA, Lingsma HF, Yoo AJ, et al. A randomized trial of intra-arterial treatment for acute ischemic stroke. N Engl J Med. 2015;372(1):11-20.
2. Goyal M, Demchuk AM, Menon BK, Eesa M, Rempel JL, Thornton J, et al. Randomized assessment of rapid endovascular treatment of ischemic stroke. N Engl J Med. 2015;372(11):1019-30.
3. Campbell BC, Mitchell PJ, Yan B, Parsons MW, Wang X, Gilligan A, et al. Endovascular therapy for ischemic stroke with perfusion-imaging selection. N Engl J Med. 2015;372(11):1009-18.
4. Abdalkader M, Siegler JE, Lee JS, Yaghi S, Qiu Z, Huo X, et al. Neuroimaging of Acute Ischemic Stroke: Multimodal Imaging Approach for Acute Endovascular Therapy. J Stroke. 2023;25(1):55-71.
5. Gao J, Parsons MW, Kawano H, Levi CR, Evans TJ, Lin L, et al. Visibility of CT early ischemic change is significantly associated with time from stroke onset to baseline scan beyond the first 3 hours of stroke onset. J Stroke. 2017;19:340-6.
6. Ko SB, Park HK, Kim BM, Heo JH, Rha JH, Kwon SU, et al. 2019 update of the Korean clinical practice guidelines of stroke for endovascular recanalization therapy in patients with acute ischemic stroke. J Stroke. 2019;21:231-40.
7. Burke JF, Kerber KA, Iwashyna TJ, Morgenstern LB. Wide variation and rising utilization of stroke magnetic resonance imaging: data from 11 states. Ann Neurol. 2012;71:179-85.
8. Brazzelli M, Sandercock PA, Chappell FM, Celani MG, Righetti E, Arestis N, et al. Magnetic resonance imaging versus computed tomography for detection of acute vascular lesions in patients presenting with stroke symptoms. Cochrane Database Syst Rev. 2009;(4):CD007424.
9. Matsumoto K, Lo EH, Pierce AR, Wei H, Garrido L, Kowall NW. Role of vasogenic edema and tissue cavitation in ischemic evolution on diffusion-weighted imaging: comparison with multiparameter MR and immunohistochemistry. AJNR Am J Neuroradiol. 1995;16:1107-15.
10. Lee SU, Hong JM, Kim SY, Bang OY, Demchuk AM, Lee JS. Differentiating carotid terminus occlusions into two distinct populations based on Willisian collateral status. J Stroke. 2016;18:179-86.
11. Rocha M, Jovin TG. Fast versus slow progressors of infarct growth in large vessel occlusion stroke: clinical and research implications. Stroke. 2017;48:2621-7.
12. Wintermark M, Sanelli PC, Albers GW, Bello J, Derdeyn C, Hetts SW, et al. Imaging recommendations for acute stroke and transient ischemic attack patients: A joint statement by the American Society of Neuroradiology, the American College of Radiology, and the Society of NeuroInterventional Surgery. AJNR Am J Neuroradiol. 2013;34(11):E117-27.
13. Cohnen M, Wittsack HJ, Assadi S, Muskalla K, Ringelstein A, Poll LW, et al. Radiation exposure of patients in comprehensive computed tomography of the head in acute stroke. AJNR Am J Neuroradiol. 2006;27:1741-5.
14. Kim JT, Cho BH, Choi KH, Park MS, Kim BJ, Park JM, et al. Magnetic resonance imaging versus computed tomography angiography based selection for endovascular therapy in patients with acute ischemic stroke. Stroke. 2019;50:365-72.

15. Alverne FJAM, Lima FO, Rocha FA, Bandeira DA, Lucena AF, Silva HC, et al. Unfavorable vascular anatomy during endovascular treatment of stroke: challenges and bailout strategies. J Stroke. 2020;22:185-202.
16. Maguida G, Shuaib A. Collateral circulation in ischemic stroke: An updated review. J Stroke. 2023;25(2):179-98.
17. Menon BK, d'Esterre CD, Qazi EM, Almekhlafi M, Hahn L, Demchuk AM, et al. Multiphase CT angiography: a new tool for the imaging triage of patients with acute ischemic stroke. Radiology. 2015;275:510-20.
18. Goyal M, Fargen KM, Turk AS, Mocco J, Liebeskind DS, Frei D, et al. Collaterals at angiography and outcomes in the Interventional Management of Stroke (IMS) III trial. Stroke. 2014;45(3):759-64.
19. Tan IY, Demchuk AM, Hopyan J, Zhang L, Gladstone D, Wong K, et al. CT angiography clot burden score and collateral score: Correlation with clinical and radiologic outcomes in acute middle cerebral artery infarct. AJNR Am J Neuroradiol. 2009;30(3):525-31.
20. Christoforidis GA, Karakasis C, Mohammad Y, Caragine LP, Yang M, Slivka A. Multimodal CT in stroke imaging: Time for a new gold standard (Pilot study evaluating the accuracy of combined/xl CT in predicting outcome of stroke patients). J Neurointerv Surg. 2009;1(2):164-8.
21. Maas MB, Lev MH, Ay H, Singhal AB, Greer DM, Smith WS, et al. Collateral vessels on CT angiography predict outcome in acute ischemic stroke. Stroke. 2009;40(9):3001-5.
22. Bang OY, Saver JL, Buck BH, Alger JR, Starkman S, Ovbiagele B, et al. Impact of collateral flow on tissue fate in acute ischaemic stroke. J Neurol Neurosurg Psychiatry. 2008;79(6):625-9.
23. Wintermark M, Albers GW, Alexandrov AV, Alger JR, Bammer R, Baron JC, et al. Delineation of the ischemic core and penumbra: Recent advances in CT perfusion imaging. J Stroke. 2020;22(1):3-10.
24. Albers GW, Marks MP, Kemp S, Christensen S, Tsai JP, Ortega-Gutierrez S, et al. Thrombectomy for stroke at 6 to 16 hours with selection by perfusion imaging. N Engl J Med. 2018;378(8):708-18.
25. Olthuis SGH, Pirson FAV, Pinckaers FME, Hinsenveld WH, Nieboer D, Ceulemans A, et al.; MR CLEAN-LATE Investigators. Endovascular treatment versus no endovascular treatment after 6-24 h in patients with ischaemic stroke and collateral flow on CT angiography (MR CLEAN-LATE) in the Netherlands: a multicentre, open-label, blinded-endpoint, randomised, controlled, phase 3 trial. Lancet. 2023;401(10385):1371-80.
26. Nogueira RG, Jadhav AP, Haussen DC, Bonafe A, Budzik RF, Bhuva P, et al. Thrombectomy 6 to 24 hours after stroke with a mismatch between deficit and infarct. N Engl J Med. 2018;378:11-21.
27. Powers WJ, Rabinstein AA, Ackerson T, Adeoye OM, Bambakidis NC, Becker K, et al. 2019 update to the 2018 Guidelines for the early management of patients with acute ischemic stroke: A guideline for healthcare professionals from the American Heart Association/American Stroke Association. Stroke. 2019;50(12):e344-e418.
28. Sarraj A, Hassan AE, Abraham MG, Ortega-Gutierrez S, Kasner SE, Hussain MS, et al. Trial of endovascular thrombectomy for large ischemic strokes. N Engl J Med. 2023;388:1259-71.
29. Huo X, Ma G, Tong X, Zhang X, Pan Y, Nguyen TN, et al. Trial of endovascular therapy for acute ischemic stroke with large infarct. N Engl J Med. 2023;388:1272-83.
30. Bendszus M, Fiehler J, Subtil F, Bonekamp S, Aamodt AH, Fuentes B, et al. Endovascular thrombectomy for acute ischaemic stroke with established large infarct: multicentre, open-label, randomised trial. Lancet. 2023;402:1753-63.
31. Zaidat OO, Kasab SA, Sheth S, Ortega-Gutierrez S, Rai AT, Given CA, et al. TESLA trial: rationale, protocol, and design. Stroke: Vasc Interv Neurol. 2023;3(4):e000787.
32. ClinicalTrials.gov. (2023). Large stroke therapy evaluation (LASTE). [online] Available from https://clinicaltrials.gov/study/NCT03811769. [Last accessed August, 2024].
33. Ji Hoe Heo, Kim K, Yoo J, Kim YD, Nam HS, Kim EY. Computed Tomography-Based Thrombus Imaging for the Prediction of Recanalization after Reperfusion Therapy in Stroke. J Stroke. 2017;19(1):40-9.
34. Menon BK. Neuroimaging in acute stroke. Continuum (Minneap Minn). 2020;26(2):287-309.
35. Kang DW, Jeong HG, Kim DY, Yang W, Lee SH. Prediction of stroke subtype and recanalization using susceptibility vessel sign on susceptibility-weighted magnetic resonance imaging. Stroke. 2017;48(6):1554-9.
36. Andrade JBC, Mohr JP, Lima FO, Barros LCM, Nepomuceno CR, Portela LB, et al. Predictors of hemorrhagic transformation after acute ischemic stroke based on the experts' opinion. Arq Neuropsiquiatr. 2021;79(4):278-85.
37. El Nawar R, Yeung J, Labreuche J, Chadenat ML, Duong DL, De Malherbe M, et al. MRI-based predictors of haemorrhagic transformation in patients with stroke treated by intravenous thrombolysis. Front Neurol. 2021;12:633712.
38. Akay EMZ, Hilbert A, Carlisle BG, Madai VI, Mutke MA, Fre D. Artificial Intelligence for Clinical Decision Support in Acute Ischemic Stroke: A Systematic Review. Stroke. 2023;54:1505-16.

Index

Page numbers followed by *f* refer to figure, and *t* refer to table.

A

Abdominal aorta 70
Abnormal uterine bleeding 92
Activated partial thromboplastin time 64, 89
Acute basilar artery occlusion 127*f*
 endovascular treatment for 52
Acute ischemic stroke 9*f*, 26, 47, 55, 57, 123, 124, 131, 132, 136*f*, 138
 management 139
 reperfusion 47
Acute left middle cerebral artery occlusion 3*f*, 4*f*
Acute stroke 1, 41, 41*t*, 134
 management 40
Alberta stroke program early computed tomography score 41, 42*f*, 126*f*, 137
Alteplase 27
 tenecteplase trial evaluation for stroke thrombolysis 30
American Heart Association 17, 86, 134, 136
American Society of Interventional and Therapeutic Neuroradiology 131
American Stroke Association 17, 35, 134, 136
Andexanet alfa 65, 66, 67*t*
Anemia 84
Aneurysm 103
Angiography 56
Angioplasty 99
Angiotensin receptor blocker 116
Anticoagulant action, reversal of 67*t*
Anticoagulation 18, 87, 87*t*
 reversal of 17
 use 16

Antiphospholipid
 antibody 85
 syndrome 119
Antithrombin deficiency 119
Antithrombotic treatment 78
Aorta 70
 abdominal 70
Aortic arch
 atheroma 70
 atherosclerosis 75*f*, 118
 axial computed tomography angiogram of 74*f*
 endarterectomy 80
 related cerebral hazard trial 78
Aortic atheroma 70, 71, 79
 grading of 72*t*
Aortic intima 73*f*
Aortic wall thickness 71*f*
Apixaban 67
Apnea-hypopnea index 117
Arch atherosclerosis, grading of 71*f*
Arterial spin labeling 132
Arterial wall 105
Artery 99*f*
 negative remodeling pattern of 99*t*
 positive remodeling pattern of 99*t*
Artificial intelligence 15, 40, 41*t*, 42*f*, 45, 139
 systems 45
Aspiration thrombectomy 54
Aspirin 7
Atherosclerosis 98, 103, 103*t*, 117
 large artery 112, 117
Atrial fibrillation 112, 118
Augmenting sonothrombolysis 5

B

Baseline intracerebral hemorrhage volume 16

Basic cardiological test 114
Basilar artery
 international cooperation study 52
 occlusion endovascular intervention 52
Behavioral modification 120
Black-hole sign 14
Blend sign 14
Blood pressure 65
 diastolic 116
 management of 65
 systolic 15, 18
Body temperature, control of 18
Brain 16, 18, 22
 computed tomography angiogram of 50*f*
 scan of 8*f*
 computer interface 43, 44
 imaging 113
 ischemia 4
 parenchyma 16
 imaging of 124
Bridging therapy 33, 33*t*, 34

C

Calcification 73, 77
Capillary index score 131
Carbonic anhydrase inhibitors 93
Cardiac rhythm monitoring 114
Cardiac tumors 119
Cardioembolism 118
Cardiomyopathy 119
Cardiovascular risk factor 9*f*
Carotid artery
 external 99
 internal 2, 98, 104, 129, 135
Carotid bifurcation 100*f*
Carotid bulb 120
 atherosclerosis of 117
Carotid endarterectomy 118
Carotid stenosis 8*f*

Carotid web 120
Catheter intra-arterial digital
    subtraction angiography 85
Cavernous sinus 84
Central nervous system 88, 101
    angiitis, primary 120
    vasculitis 101
Cerebellar hemisphere 127*f*
Cerebral amyloid angiopathy 12
Cerebral artery 97
    anterior 2-4, 51, 104
    middle 3, 8, 9, 41, 48, 52, 99,
        104, 127, 129, 133, 135
    posterior 51
Cerebral blood
    flow 43, 132, 133
    volume 132, 133
Cerebral circulation failure, type
    of 112
Cerebral collateral circulation
    130*t*
Cerebral infarction 52
    score 54
Cerebral microbleeds 35
Cerebral venous thrombosis 83,
    87, 89, 89*t*, 90, 92
    management of 83, 89*f*
Cerebrospinal fluid 86, 97
Cholesterol 101
    esters 101
Clopidogrel 7
Common carotid artery 99
Computed tomography 50, 78
    angiography 2, 13, 15, 50*f*, 51,
        70, 75, 96, 128, 129, 131
    perfusion 52, 131
        imaging 31
        protocol of 132
Contact aspiration 54
Continuous positive airway
    pressure 117
Contrast-enhanced
    magnetic resonance angiogram
        76*f*
    perfusion 132
Convolutional neural networks
    43
Cortical vein 84
Corticosteroids 84
COVID-19 84, 90, 94
    infection 112
    vaccine 85, 92

D

Dash diet 115
Decompression craniectomy 20,
    93
Deep learning 40
Deep venous
    system 84
    thrombosis 62
Dehydration 84, 90
Depression 21
Diabetes 116
Diet 114
Diffusion-weighted imaging 48,
    126, 127, 135, 136
Digital subtraction angiography
    85, 124, 130
    techniques 96
Direct aspiration first pass
    technique 54
Direct endovascular therapy 33*t*,
    34
Direct-acting oral anticoagulants
    61-63, 65*t*, 87-89, 120
    action
        after reversal, resumption
            of 68
        assessment of 64
    reversal of 65
    management of 61
Distal medium vessel occlusions
    50
Distal vessels 51
Dolichoectasia 120
Dural arteriovenous fistula 90
Dynamic susceptibility contrast
    perfusion 132

E

Eccentricity 101
Echocardiography 72
Echoplanar imaging thrombolytic
    evaluation trial 28
Elastic lamina, internal 97
Elastic membranes, external 98
Electrocardiogram 113
Electrocardiography 77
Elevated intracranial pressure,
    management of 93
Embolic stroke 112, 120
Emergency neurological deficits 28

Encephalopathy 120
End-diastolic velocity 8
Endovascular therapy 1, 30, 47,
    49, 50, 52, 53, 135-137, 139
    techniques 54
Endovascular thrombectomy 6
Endovascular treatment,
    theoretical advantages of 92
Epiaortic echocardiography 79
Epiaortic ultrasound 74
European Cooperative Acute
    Stroke Study 27, 48
European Stroke Organisation
    15, 85
Extracranial atherosclerosis 117
Extracranial vessels 96
    imaging of 128

F

Fabry's disease 108
Factor V Leiden mutation 119
Fibromuscular dysplasia 120
Fibrous cap 101
Fibrous tissue 77
Fluid-attenuated inversion
    recovery 127, 128, 135, 136
Fluid-blood level 14
Fluorine 78
Fluorodeoxyglucose 78
French Study on Aortic Plaques in
    Stroke 71
Fresh frozen plasma 65
Fusiform dilatation 120

G

Gemstone spectral imaging 15
Genetic testing 86
Glasgow coma scale 18
Glucose analogue 78
Glycemic control 18
Gradient echo 128

H

Head trauma 90
Headache 88
    severe acute 102
Health system-based intervention
    120
Heart

disease
  congenital 119
  valvular 118
  rate 8
Hematoma
  expansion 13, 13t, 15, 21
  surgical evacuation of 17
Hemodialysis 66
Hemorrhage 77
  anticoagulant associated 63
  detection 41
  fatal 61
  intracerebral 13, 16, 18, 21, 61, 63
  intracranial 32, 42, 87, 89
  intraplaque 101
  intraventricular 18
  major 61
Hemorrhagic avalanche 16
Hemorrhagic transformation
  assessment of 126
  predictors of 139
Heparin, unfractionated 87, 89
High-flow velocity 100
High-resolution
  intracranial vessel wall magnetic resonance imaging 96
  vascular wall imaging 96
Hounsfield units 15
Hydrophilic necrosis 77
Hypercoagulable state 119
Hyperhomocysteinemia 119
Hyperlipidemia 78, 116
Hypertension 12, 116
Hypertriglyceridemia 116
Hypoperfusion
  infract 113
  partial 52f
Hypoxia 90

I

Idarucizumab 65, 66
Infarct core, quantification of 132t
International normalized ratio 18, 27, 87, 89
Intracerebral hemorrhage 13, 16, 18, 21, 61, 63
  surgical management of 19
  symptomatic 5, 27, 48, 137

Intracranial arteriosclerotic disease 98
Intracranial atherosclerosis 117
Intracranial atherosclerotic disease 101, 103, 104, 124
  stenosis 138
    predictors of 138
Intracranial hemorrhage 32, 42, 87, 89
  detection 42f
  identification 42
Intracranial stenting 56
Intracranial vessels 96
  imaging of 128
Intraplaque hemorrhage 101
Intravenous thrombolysis 4f, 26, 47, 135, 136, 139
  therapy 35
Intraventricular extension 16
Iodine sign 14
Ischemia, cerebral 113
Ischemic stroke 49
  early detection of 126
  rapid endovascular treatment of 123
Island sign 14

L

Lactic acidosis 120
Lacunar 112
Lacunar strokes, identification of 126
Large core acute ischemic stroke 53
Large deep supratentorial intracerebral hemorrhages 20
Large vessel occlusion 3, 30, 41, 49, 54, 57, 124, 134, 136
  detection 41, 42f
L-asparaginase 84
Leakage sign 13
Left ventricular thrombus 119
Lemierre syndrome 90
Linear atheroma 71f
Lipid core 101
Lipid-rich core 77
Low National Institute of Health Stroke Scale, endovascular therapy for 49
Low-density lipoprotein 116
  cholesterol 79

Low-flow velocity 100
Low-intensity electromagnetic fields 44
Low-molecular weight heparin 87, 89

M

Maas collateral score 131
Machine learning 15, 40
Magnetic resonance
  angiographic techniques 128
  angiography 2, 51, 96, 128, 130
  imaging 31, 48, 70, 76, 77, 79, 85, 96, 101, 125
  perfusion 132
Malignancy 120
Mastoiditis 90
Mean flow velocity 3
Mean transit time 52, 132, 133
Mechanical thrombectomy 6, 47, 123, 136t
Meningitis 90
Microembolic signals 7
Minimally invasive surgery 18, 19
Mitochondrial myopathy 120
Mobile thrombus 73
Moyamoya disease 103, 103t, 104, 118
Multiphase computed tomography angiography 130

N

National Institute of Health Stroke Scale 2, 3f, 8, 9, 49, 50, 52, 64
National Institute of Neurological Disorders and Stroke 26
Negative predictive value 15
Neuroparenchyma, ischemic 127f
Nonatherosclerotic diseases 101, 120
Noncontrast computed tomography 15, 125-127, 129, 135, 137
  scan 21
Norwegian Tenecteplase Stroke Trial 30
Novel oral anticoagulant 19
Nutrition 114

O

Obesity 94, 117
Obstructive sleep apnea 117

P

Paradoxical embolism 9f
Parenchyma 133
Patent foramen ovale 9, 119
Penetrating atherosclerotic ulcer 79
Penumbra 132t
Percutaneous transluminal angioplasty 117
Plaque
  content 101, 101f
  formation 99
    mechanism of 100f
  morphology 73
  thrombosis 73
Plasminogen activator inhibitor-1 28
Positive predictive value 15
Positron emission tomography 70, 78
Posterior circulation large vessel occlusion, endovascular therapy for 51
Posterior communication artery 3
Posterior fossa strokes, evaluation of 126
Post-intracerebral hemorrhages care 20
Pregnancy 91
Protein
  C deficiency 119
  S deficiency 119
Prothrombin
  complex concentrate 18, 65
  time 89
Puerperium 91
Pulsatility index 8

R

Raised intracranial pressure, management of 93
Randomized controlled trial 27, 53
Rankin scale, modified 27, 30, 34, 54
Recanalization 94
Recombinant tissue plasminogen activator 26, 27, 31, 32
Recurrent ischemic stroke study 78
Regional leptomeningeal collateral score 131
Rehabilitation 41, 43
Reperfusion therapies 92
Resistance index 8
Respiratory infections 84
Reversible cerebral vasoconstriction syndrome 102-104
Rheumatic heart disease 118
Rivaroxaban 67
  oral 91
Robotics 41
Routine blood parameter 114

S

Salvageable brain tissue 48
Satellite sign 14
Seizures 88
Sepsis 84
Sickle cell disease 120
Sigmoid sinus 84
Single antiplatelet therapy 118
Sinotubular junction 70
Sinus thrombosis 84t
Small strokes, identification of 126
Small vessel disease 15, 21, 112, 117, 118
Society of Interventional Radiology 131
Sonothrombolysis 5
Special blood tests 114
Spontaneous intracerebral hemorrhage 12
  treatment of 16
Spot sign 13, 15
Steno-occlusive diseases 104f, 105f
Stent-retriever thrombectomy 54
Stroke 26, 47, 49, 83, 111, 120
  acute 1, 41, 41t, 134
  classification of 12t, 112t
  diagnostic evaluation of 112
  embolic 112, 120
  hemorrhagic 61
  hyperacute ischemic 2, 3
  ischemic 49
  mechanism of 100, 112
  mimics, assessment of 126
  minor 35
  nonlacunar cryptogenic embolic pattern of 120
  pathophysiology of 112, 113f
  posterior circulation 127f, 130f
  prevention 7
  recurrent 119
  secondary prevention of 111, 112
  terminology 112
  type 112
  wake-up 48
Subarachnoid extension 13, 14
Substance abuse 115
Superior sagittal sinus 84
Swirl sign 14
Symptomatic carotid stenosis 7
Syncope 113

T

T1-weighted imaging 77
Tamoxifen 84
Tan collateral score 131
Tandem lesions 8
Telestroke 56
Tenecteplase 28, 31, 32, 48
  dose of 31
  efficacy of 31
Thalidomide 84
Thoracic aorta 70
Threatened morphology 99
Thrombectomy 54, 105
Thrombin time 63
Thrombocytopenia
  effect of 105
  vaccine-induced 94
Thrombolysis 4, 52
  modified 54
Thrombolytic drug 48
Thrombosis 91
Thrombus characterization 138
Time-of-flight 128, 130
Tissue plasminogen activator 3
Topiramate 93
Tranexamic acid 19
Transcranial Doppler 1-4, 8, 9, 114
  emboli detection 7
  role of 6, 7
  therapeutic role of 5
Transcranial ultrasound 6
Transesophageal echocardiography 9, 70, 72, 73f, 79, 114

Transient ischemic attack 78, 112, 113
Transthoracic echocardiography 72
Transverse sinus 84
Triglyceride 101
Tumor necrosis factor 100

U

Ulceration 73
Ultrasound contrast agents 5
Vaccine-induced immune thrombotic thrombocytopenia 92
Valsalva maneuver 9

Vasa vasorum 97, 105
  externa 97
  interna 97
Vascular imaging 114
  modalities 1
Vascular malformations 15
Vascular reversible angiographic abnormalities 102
Vascular risk factor management 114
Vasculitis 103*t*, 104, 120
Venous thromboembolism 87
Venous thrombosis 91
Ventricular drainage, external 17, 18

Vertebrobasilar segment, tortuosity of 120
Vessel wall 75
  magnetic resonance imaging
    pitfalls of 105
    protocol of 97
    sequences for 97
  pathologies 104*t*
Visual loss 90
Vitamin K antagonist 18, 63, 87, 89

W

Wake-up strokes 48
Willis circle 130